Implementation

THE 20 BILLION DOLLAR DIET ®

fiber — 25 grams/day — 40/6 to loose wt. per si
protein — 45 grams/day
fat — 50 grams

THE 20 BILLION DOLLAR DIET ®

Why diets fail and how to lose weight for good

Marina MacDonald, M.S., Ph.D. and Judith A. McManus, M.A.

ISBN-13: 9781532704383
ISBN-10: 1532704380
Library of Congress Control Number: 2016906207
CreateSpace Independent Publishing Platform
North Charleston, South Carolina

The information included in this book is for educational purposes only. It is not intended nor implied to be a substitute for professional medical, nutritional, or psychological advice or treatment. The reader should consult his or her healthcare provider before starting any diet or exercise program, to determine the appropriateness of the information for their own situation, and to address any concerns or questions they may have regarding any medical condition or health problem. Neither the authors nor the publisher shall be liable or responsible for any loss or damage allegedly arising from any information or suggestion in this book.

The 20 Billion Dollar Diet® is a registered trademark of Marina MacDonald and Judith A. McManus.

Table of Contents

Introduction

The significant problems we have cannot be solved
at the same level of thinking with which we created them.
~ ALBERT EINSTEIN

Americans spend more than \$20 billion annually for weight loss plans, books, supplements and "fat-burning foods." Still, according to a Gallup poll, the obesity rate is higher than ever. More than half of Americans say they are trying to drop some weight, but fewer than one in five individuals succeed. A survey of over 50 million overweight Americans who tried to lose weight showed that, instead of losing, the average dieter *gained* almost five pounds in a single year. America is on a \$20 billion diet that isn't working!

Dieting used to be part of my life. Name a diet and I'll bet that I've been on it at least once, maybe two or even three times. Like many Americans, I've spent thousands of dollars on weight-loss consultations, programs, physicians, pills, formulas, DVDs, lectures, web conferences, and best-selling books about achieving and maintaining a healthy weight. You and I may have purchased some of the same self-help books, taking comfort that we could lose 20 pounds in 20 days, cleanse our bodies and souls in 21 days, or be thin forever if only we followed a plan designed by a diet guru.

I've tried lots of popular diet plans: no carbs, all carbs, points and point-free foods, all liquid, prepackaged, and so on and so forth. Before I was married, a friend and I went to a physician who specialized in liquid diets so that we could emulate Oprah when she lost weight on a medically-supervised plan. And with another friend, I found a second physician who prescribed pills and a diet centered on animal protein. I rationalized all of the expenditures by telling myself that if I spent money for a diet guru's plan, I'd be more inclined to keep the weight off forever.

Unfortunately, my old strategies and expenditures never resulted in long-term fitness and weight loss. It seems that I could follow an author, physician, or weight-loss-company's plan and lose about ten to twenty pounds. Then stress, cravings, and old habits would resurface and I'd be back to combining junk food with little physical exercise. Inevitably, I'd gain even more weight. I crowned myself as a yo-yo queen.

Like me, many of you have outsourced your diet to others, thus fueling a multi-billion-dollar market for weight loss products and services. Unless Americans implement an entirely new paradigm and strategies, we will continue to waste money on diets that fail.

About 50 pounds ago, my life changed. I'd finally had it, and I mean *really* had it with yo-yo dieting, wearing long tops that covered my hips and most of my thighs, avoiding scales, and truly not living the life I envisioned. I wanted to gain control, avoid temptation, and stop overeating and binge-ing. I simply asked myself, "Are you happy with the way you look and feel?" When I answered "No," I knew it was time to make some changes. Maya Angelou's saying, "The need to change bulldozed a path through my mind," resonated loudly and clearly in my psyche. I *had* to eliminate the pounds and the emotional baggage that was figuratively and literally weighing me down.

Recognizing that outsourcing was not the solution to my problem, I decided that I would no longer pay for another weight loss plan. I was tired of delegating my diet to individuals or corporations who supposedly knew more about my habits, preferences, and health than I did. Empowerment began when I recognized that I needed to investigate what foods, coping strategies, and long-term plan were best *for me*. This book is based on a vision, a plan, and a desire to find my inner truth and maximize my physical health. You can do the same.

The first truth that emerged from my journey is that most diets fail because they provide a top-down, one-size-fits-all, externally-prescribed approach to losing weight. When I stopped outsourcing, took complete ownership for my health, and created a holistic plan that was *internally right for me*, I was successful.

Importantly, most diets fail because they fail to address the internal and external forces that promote overeating. Thus, as soon as the official diet ends, the weight comes back on. This book illuminates these universal forces from the standpoint of physiology and psychology, and provides specific strategies and tactics to put YOU back in the driver's seat, so that you can lose weight once and for all.

With Marina, I was able to understand the scientific basis of overeating. Together with our knowledge and skills as an educator and a scientist, we have combined my personal journey and experience with cutting-edge studies of appetite and human behavior to illuminate ten scientific principles for achieving and maintaining a healthy weight. We've integrated research and professional advice with practical experience so that you can achieve your goals for good.

In *The 20 Billion Dollar Diet*® you'll learn how the cards are stacked against those of us who have weight issues in our obesogenic environment, an environment that encourages overeating and promotes obesity. We'll examine these forces as well as how to overcome them. You'll understand the role of your own history and emotions and the importance of external and internal cues that conspire to keep us overweight. Throughout the book you'll focus on proven strategies and tactics to achieve your weight goal, and you'll be an active participant in your own plan by completing guided exercises at the end of each chapter. One of the many exciting parts about what we've written is that the information is all documented by scientific studies, which are listed in the Scientific Citations section and indexed to phrases in the text. Know that transforming your body and health is a complex yet understandable and totally manageable process that you can master.

If you're tired of being overweight and you're ready to transform your body and your life, you're in the right place. Armed with the knowledge in this book, you too can achieve the goal weight you have wanted for so long.

1

Believe and Commit

Almost all successful people begin with two beliefs:
The future can be better than the present,
and I have the power to make it so.
~ David Brooks, *New York Times* Columnist

The first step to losing weight is *to believe* that you will lose weight. Sounds hokey? Kind of. Sounds simple enough? It is. Unfortunately, many people begin dieting with a halfhearted belief that maybe, just maybe, some magic will take place and fat will disappear. And then there are many people who stay on a diet for a few weeks and if results aren't fast enough, it's back to old eating patterns. I've been there and done that. Nothing lost. Nothing gained, except more weight.

Achieving and maintaining your weight goal doesn't happen by invoking "maybes" or magical thinking. It involves a process of change which takes us outside of our comfort zone. Change requires that we leave behind habits that are comfortable even if they are not meeting our goals.

There were many times that I "tried out" diets and "hoped" that one would work forever. When I finally felt and expressed, "Enough is enough," "The costs outweigh the rewards," and "I can do this," I was unstoppable. An important aspect of commitment is weighing the pros and cons of both the problem and the solution. Once I did this, I recognized that the costs of being overweight far surpassed the rewards.

There's a great deal of power in making a commitment, believing that you can succeed, and sticking to it. Know that the past does not equal the future and that by truly committing to a change of lifestyle, you are guaranteeing your chance of success. Embrace the process of change and remind yourself that you can accomplish whatever you set your mind on.

Mindsets are just beliefs.
They're powerful beliefs, but they're just something
in your mind,
and you can change your mind.
~ Dr. Carol S. Dweck

Your own belief in your ability to complete tasks and reach your goals is called *self-efficacy* and it is a top predictor of success. According to psychologist Albert Bandura, self-efficacy plays a major role in how we approach tasks, challenges, and goals. You may believe in yourself more now than ever before, or like many of us, you may have experienced so many failures in dieting that you're not sure of your own ability. If we believe that we will perform well, we are more apt to view difficult tasks as something to be mastered rather than something to be avoided. Henry Ford's quotation is applicable to building self-efficacy, "Whether you believe you can do a thing or not, you are right."

Many people cite a lack of willpower as a reason for not achieving their goals to lose weight. Dr. Carol Dweck, author of *Mindset: The New Psychology of Success*, posits that willpower can indeed be quite limited – but only if you believe it is. Studies by Dweck and colleagues have shown that when people believed their willpower was limited, they acted accordingly, for example by eating more junk food when they were in a stressful situation. Under the same circumstances, people who believed their willpower was *not* limited ate *less* junk food than their colleagues.

Additional studies have shown that your belief in yourself can be enhanced by repeating a simple implementation intention, also known as an if-then plan, like this one: "If I encounter a problem, then I will tell myself: *I can solve this challenge.*" Another effective strategy for dealing with temptation is to view the situation as a personal challenge with an immediate goal: *to prove that you have willpower.*

It's been proven that through the use of simple practices such as establishing goals and monitoring your behavior as well as reframing your thoughts, you can increase your belief in yourself, redirect your behaviors, and rewire your brain. You'll practice these strategies throughout this book.

> *The only thing that stands between a person and*
> *what they want in life*
> *is the will to try it*
> *and the faith to believe it is possible.*
> ~Richard DeVos

It's also interesting to note that weight-loss success is not necessarily a function of willpower. In fact, people with high self-control may use their willpower *less* often than the rest of us, by proactively avoiding situations that could challenge their self-control. This discovery puts the weight-loss challenge in a whole new light. It means that some of the most effective weight-loss tactics are those that *reduce the need for willpower*. For example, by formulating a plan to avoid high-sugar/high-fat foods and triggers, we can minimize conflicts between temptations and weight-loss goals. These and other smart tactics can be practiced, along with healthy eating, until they become habits.

It may seem magical, but believing in your abilities actually shifts neural responses that can open our minds to positive change. An understanding of the biological basis of overeating gives us the strategies we need to change our approach. And persistence – simply carrying on in the face of challenges or setbacks - impels more positive change. Be your own advocate and cheerleader and *know* that you will succeed.

IMPLEMENTATION

Believe and Commit is the first scientific principle of weight-loss success. If you believe and commit, you can accomplish more than you ever thought possible.

Reflect on your answers to the following questions. They'll provide valuable information about your current and future behaviors.

1. Write down a few words to describe your weight: fat, overweight, obese, heavy, unbearable, nice size, etc.
2. What words do you wish you could use to describe your body?
3. What's holding you back from eating healthy meals and losing weight?
4. Consider your mindset. Do you believe that your behavior is fixed (immutable) or do you believe that it can be changed through experimentation and practice? Write down some examples of challenges you have successfully tackled in the past. Are you willing to view weight loss as a challenge that you can tackle?
5. Create a list of costs and rewards of maintaining your current weight and eating habits. Use our *Costs and Rewards of Being Overweight* table as a model. Consider various costs of being overweight, such as: *It's harder to move, I feel less confident*, or *I am jeopardizing my health*.

COSTS & REWARDS

COSTS of being overweight	REWARDS of being overweight
Being overweight or obese can increase the risk for diabetes, heart disease, cancer, gallstones, and osteoarthritis.*	Temporarily, hyperpalatable foods can get your mind off of tasks, stressors, and problems.
My high cholesterol is associated with excess weight.	Many hyperpalatable processed foods have strong, attractive tastes for all parts of your tongue.
I am not able to participate in a 5K run.	I receive compliments for baking high-sugar/high-fat foods, and I can't bake without eating.
My doctor recommends weight loss.	There is a sense of reward when you can eat whatever you want.

*National Institutes of Health (NIH)

6. Analyze your responses to items 1-5. Now answer the following questions. Do you *believe* that you will accomplish your goal? Do you *commit* 100% to losing weight? If you *believe* that the time has come to create change, *commit* to being fit.

2

Tell Your Story

*I believe that half the unhappiness in life comes from
people being afraid to go straight at things.*
~ WILLIAM J. LOCKE

In order to get a handle on my relationship with food, I began by examining my family history and background. I grew up in the Midwest and our family meals consisted of well-balanced, hearty foods such as fried chicken, roast beef, lamb chops, salad, grains, and vegetables. We grew delicious tomatoes, lettuce, and cucumbers in a garden and we had a couple of fruit trees that supplied fresh organic pears and apples. Potatoes or bread accompanied a typical meal of meat, vegetables, and a salad or coleslaw. Dairy milk was my beverage of choice and I could easily drink four to five glasses of whole milk per day.

I don't remember eating dessert with lunch or dinner, but I do remember eating cake, candy, and other "treats" between meals. At least once a week, my mother and I baked and ate sweets such as chocolate cake, brownies, chocolate chip cookies, or cherry pies. I have many special memories of baking, laughing, and eating. School or parties and holidays always involved eating a lot of high-sugar/high-fat foods at school, home, and friends' houses. As a result, like many people who struggle with their weight, I grew up associating candy, cake, chips, and cookies with comfort, fun, and rewards. This reinforced my habit of consuming such foods whenever I felt that I needed or deserved a reward. Much later, I would see the light and develop a more accurate equation demonstrating that high-sugar/high-fat foods are the *antithesis* of rewards.

Sugar + Fat ≠ Reward

Although I ate hearty meals and enjoyed sweets in my youth, food was primarily a source of energy for all of my activities. I was physically active as I loved swimming, biking, dancing, roller skating, and softball. I was about average in height and bone structure, well proportioned, athletic, and didn't have a problem with my weight throughout my childhood. Some time in my teens, I noticed that models and actresses were extremely thin and my vision of what was a normal size changed accordingly. I began skipping breakfast and by mid-morning I was starving. Hungry and in a hurry to get to class, I purchased candy bars or some other junk food to tide me over until lunch.

By skipping breakfast and then indulging in sugary junk food, I was setting myself up for a lifetime of weight struggles. Food restriction intensifies the desire for sugar and can precipitate food cravings, binge eating, and obesity. Researchers recently discovered a specific neural circuit that controls compulsive sugar consumption, which demonstrates that there really is a pathway to compulsion. Animals can be turned into binge-eaters by depriving them of food for 12 hours and then offering them sugar water along with their normal chow. Soon they begin to escalate their daily intake of sugar and to gulp it down in a binge-like fashion. After a few weeks of bingeing, animals show adaptations in the brain that are similar to changes seen with addictive drugs. These studies demonstrate that binge eating has a neurochemical basis and that sugar is a big part of the problem. Meal skipping leads to a greater desire for sugar which in turn leads to overeating as demonstrated in the following formula.

Fasting and/or meal skipping → ↑ desire for sugar
→ overeating and/or binge eating

Toward the end of my senior year in high school, a friend and I decided that we needed to lose weight so we fasted for a few days and then "rewarded" our weight loss by eating a three-layer cake. I'm pretty sure that my habit of bingeing began with that "diet." In college, another friend and I decided that a four-day diet of rice and apple juice, followed by saunas, was a terrific way to cleanse our systems while losing weight. Once again, after we completed the diet and lost 10 pounds, most of which was probably water loss, our "reward" was an all-you-can-eat buffet.

EMOTIONAL TRIGGERS AND OVEREATING

Looking back at my past, I realized that certain emotional triggers often resulted in overeating. When I wasn't on an official diet or a plan pre-scribed by a book, company, or weight-loss physician, I would overeat when I faced difficult emotional situations. When I engaged in overeating, I disregarded nutrition, eating a lot of high-sugar/high-fat food in a short period of time when I wasn't always physically hungry.

Binge eating involves recurrent episodes of eating an abnormally large amount of food and feeling a lack of control over food. I have friends who eat bags of candy, chips, and soda at work and I've binged on comfort foods when faced with unpleasant emotions. The official diagnostic criteria for Binge Eating Disorder include bingeing at least once a week over a period of at least three months. Even if binge eating occurs less frequently, it is a problem for many individuals.

One important point is that there is a spectrum of overeating behav-iors, ranging from mild to severe. Some of us engage in passive overeat-ing, eating a little too much over a long period of time. Others experience episodes of out-of-control or binge eating. Although I was never officially diagnosed with an eating disorder, I still experienced overeating.

When faced with stress or challenges, I often ate chips, candy, and pas-tries in an attempt to cope. A normal size of anything just wasn't enough and if I was going to pig out, my foods of choice would be high in fat and sugar. I'm not alone in my preferences, as research tells us that binge-eat-ing episodes often involve chocolate, ice cream, and other hyperpalatable foods. The word *hyperpalatable* is coined from the prefix hyper-, "excessive"; and palatable, "pleasing to the sense of taste."

My overeating involved eating after I was full. I didn't want to know how many calories I was consuming as I mindlessly acted on a compulsion. A compulsion is an irresistible impulse to act regardless of the rationality of the motivation. For many people, a pattern of frequent compulsive overeating is similar to what is understood by terms like substance abuse. While compulsive eating of sugary foods may not be as life-disruptive as heroin or cocaine use, it may be far more pervasive.

Despite all the crazy dieting, I maintained a relatively normal weight until I hit the "sandwich generation" of people who care for their aging parents while supporting their own children. Like many single women, I was not taking care of myself. I yo-yoed and then succumbed to a major weight gain as I maneuvered through life's challenges, trying to play the best game with the hand I was dealt. My life challenges were similar to ones that everyone experiences, and no one is a victim in life. We all make choices and react to external and internal demands to the best of our abilities at any one time.

For many of us, intensely sweet foods create a dependence on sugar. The word *dependence* means "the state of relying on or being controlled by someone or something else." Approximately 20% of obese individuals meet the criteria for a substance use disorder according to pioneering studies by Dr. Ashley Gearhardt and colleagues at Yale University. A loss of control over food consumption, continued overeating despite negative consequences, and an inability to cut down on food intake are some of the symptoms assessed in the Yale Food Addiction Survey, which is modeled after the criteria for substance dependence. Binge Eating Disorder is most closely linked with high scores on the Yale Food Addiction Survey.

The feeling of loss of control over food, or any other substance, is not pleasurable. The problem with bingeing - and all addictions for that matter - is that you are never satisfied. You want more and more and before you know it, the thrill is gone. At first, a little is not enough and then after a while a lot is not enough. Not surprisingly, overeating can mask emotions and exacerbate one's inability to cope.

The feeling of guilt, and shame for many overeaters, is a direct result of the sense of loss of control that accompanies addictive behaviors including binge eating, smoking, and alcohol and drug abuse. Shame is a particularly unproductive emotion that keeps us stuck and feeling powerless. If you tend to view overeating as a moral failure or a character flaw, you may be prone to experiencing shame about your eating along with the sense that you are unable to alter your behavior. To move beyond shame, keep in mind that animals – *which do not have moral failings* – also overeat under conditions that simulate obesogenic environments, especially where sugar is involved.

In our opinion, the evidence that overeating has a biological rather than a moral explanation provides us with the freedom to tackle the problem in our own lives. Rather than becoming mired in self-criticism, we can ditch the feelings of guilt and shame and actively explore ways to take control of the situation.

THE RELATIONSHIP BETWEEN DIET AND EXERCISE

When I wasn't on an official diet, my physical activity level was usually sedentary. Typically, I was working at least eight hours per day at a computer, handling day-to-day responsibilities, and organizing carpools, meals, and other tasks. I figured that even a 30 minute period of exercise was impossible in my overly taxed and stressful schedule.

As I contemplate my heavier days, I can see the strong correlation between a lack of exercise and unhealthy eating. Whenever I am inactive I tend to eat more high-sugar/high-fat foods and have less energy. When I was eating a lot of high-sugar/high-fat food, I didn't feel like walking or hiking or biking. Eat a bag of chips, a burger and a brownie, and see if you feel like walking briskly for an hour. I'll be surprised if you do. On the other hand, if you have a nutritious salad, whole grain bread, and a piece of fruit, you probably could walk a mile or more. Nutritious foods boost energy while high-sugar/high-fat foods weigh us down.

Now I know that if I eat nutritious food, cut out junk food, and exercise more, my perception of myself and life are more positive and I am better equipped to enjoy life's blessings as well as to reframe challenges. In my heavier days, I unconsciously and sometimes consciously ignored *why* I was overeating as well as what I ate. It's symbolic that that I would write one-page diary entries about my weight and then carelessly stuff them in cardboard boxes. Out of sight, out of mind.

I looked at myself in the mirror from the neck up and made sure that I was always standing in the back when group photos were taken. Shopping presented problems, but I relied on loose-fitting clothes, elasticized waist bands, and the color black. Along with dressing to conceal my weight during my "sandwich" years, I told myself that I could change my habits any time that I wanted to. I'd remember my high school and college days when I was able to lose ten pounds in a couple of weeks by following a quick weight-loss diet.

My common justifications for overeating were that I deserved a reward for working ten hours or that I could overeat because the next day I'd start a new diet. I now know that I am not alone as justifications are commonly used by people who overeat despite wanting to lose weight. It is human nature to protect our egos by defending our actions to ourselves. However, justifications undermine our weight-loss goals by providing a *de facto* license to overeat.

It's not surprising that justifications have wormed their way into food advertising. For example, the top advertising jingle of the 20th Century was "You deserve a break today." The slogan's creator said that part of the power of the ad was that the phrase "You deserve" *granted consumers permission* to indulge in a meal at the hamburger chain. Most of us are unaware that these seemingly innocuous messages work at a subconscious level to promote overeating.

It takes a deliberate effort to change thoughts, habits, and responses that have persisted for years. The good news is that by addressing your eating patterns and habits head-on, you'll move one step closer to solving your weight-loss challenge.

STOP SEEKING AN ESCAPE THROUGH FOOD

When we stop seeking an escape through food, we are more inclined to take an active role in life's rewards as well as to develop healthy coping mechanisms for the inevitable setbacks of life. The task of becoming mindful and re-tooling our behaviors is both complex and yet 100% possible, empowering, and exciting. A weight loss strategy that takes into account our biological requirements for nutritious food, activity, sleep, and relief of stress will help us to succeed. I am living testament of our ability to take charge, change our thinking, and alter our life course. It's powerful and true that you are equipped and able to do the same.

IMPLEMENTATION

An important tenet of *The 20 Billion Dollar Diet* is that losing weight has a lot more to do with your mind, feelings, and emotions than just plain food. Behaviors can quickly become habits and the more times you repeat the habit, the stronger the neural path and the more automatic the behavior becomes.

Tell Your Story is the second scientific principle of weight-loss success. Through awareness, you can redirect negative behavior and reprogram new and positive behaviors. Understanding your past will help you to improve your present.

In this exercise, dig deep into your relationship with food. Write from your heart and mind. You may want to reread my story in order to reflect on your past and write your own narrative.

1. Looking back on your childhood and school years, can you identify habits that began in your youth which still persist today?
2. Did family members model healthy or unhealthy behaviors for you?
3. Were "treats" given as rewards, or withheld as punishment? Be as specific as possible as you recall the influences of your environment on your current food choices, habits, and behaviors.
4. When was the first time that you knew you were overweight? How long ago was that?
5. What is your eating pattern (eating over the period of one week)? Calories? Types of foods?
6. What diets have you been on? Discuss the positives and negatives with the diets.
7. Do you overeat? What time of day? In what situations?
8. Do you eat and/or overeat to deal with difficult emotions? Explain.
9. If you overeat, what foods, special events, stressors, or feelings (anxiety, tension, boredom, or loneliness) are triggers? What will you do to reframe these triggers?

10. Discuss your history with physical exercise. What activities did you enjoy as a youth?

11. What types of physical activity do you get each day? Are there any forms of physical activity that you'd like to participate in but are not able to due to your weight? How does your diet affect your physical activity? Use the *Relationship between Diet and Exercise* table to analyze your own lifestyle.

RELATIONSHIP BETWEEN DIET and EXERCISE

Has the cycle on the left manifested in your life? If so, you're like most overweight individuals.

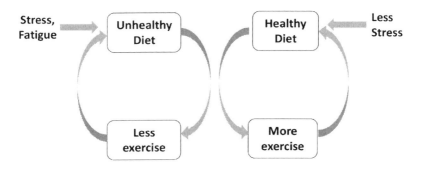

We prefer the healthy diet & exercise cycle on the right. And you?

12. Analyze your responses to items #1-11. Take special note of your 1) eating patterns, 2) overeating triggers and foods, 3) reframing and redirecting responses to triggers, 4) current exercise level, and 5) future exercise plans.

3

Our Obesogenic Environment

*A more accurate conceptualization of the obesity epidemic
is that people are responding to the forces in their environment,
rather than lacking in willpower and self-control.*
~ Dr. Deborah A. Cohen, author of *A Big Fat Crisis*

Scientific research reveals that there is much, much more to overeating, bingeing, and unhealthy food choices than just liking food. The first step is to understand what is triggering our behaviors. My own issues and habits are rooted in our modern obesogenic environment, unhealthy levels of stress, and excessive quantities of high-sugar/high-fat foods. If we become aware of these forces, and the way in which they promote overeating, we can begin to reverse the trend in our own lives.

One of the most eye-opening truths about my own eating, and our society in general, is that our environment *promotes* excessive weight gain and *produces* obesity. As the Harvard School of Public Health says, "The world in which most consumers live makes choosing healthy food *very hard* and choosing unhealthy food *very easy* [emphasis added]. It's truly a toxic environment that eats away at healthy lifestyles and promotes obesity."

Between 1970 and 2000, our average calorie consumption increased by a whopping 530 calories per person per day. Calorie intake has increased because of more available, cheap, tasty, obesogenic foods. How interesting that the obesity epidemic paralleled the availability and promotion of junk foods including sugary sodas, chips, cookies, pastries and other ultra- processed foods, which now account for nearly 60% of calories along with 90% of the sugar we consume. The calories in these foods are known as "empty calories" because they add to calorie intake without providing essential nutrients such as vitamins or minerals.

At the same time, we are not eating enough nutrient-dense foods to meet U.S. guidelines for healthy diets. The term "nutrient-dense" refers to foods that are high in nutrients and relatively low in calories. Nutrient-dense foods can be found in the five major food groups: vegetables, fruits, whole grains, healthy protein sources and low-fat milk products, all of which are important for good health and weight control. On average, less than one-third of our calories come from nutrient-dense, unprocessed foods.

A lack of physical activity is part of the obesogenic equation. Fifty years ago, we were moderately active as a population. Now, our work and home environments are largely sedentary. Although we *need* fewer calories at home and at work, we are consuming *more*. Unlike our ancestors, we do not need to expend any energy hunting or gathering food unless we happen to be farmers, ranchers, or mountain people on a reality TV show. To quantify the impact of sedentary behaviors on weight gain, the Nurses' Health Study followed more than 50,000 middle-age women for six years to look at behaviors such as watching television. Women who watched television for two hours each day had, on average, a 23 percent increased risk of becoming obese. Not only do we eat more food when it is hyperpalatable, but we eat more of such foods when we are sedentary.

A lack of sleep is strongly associated with hunger, overeating, and weight gain. Over the last 50 years, the amount of sleep Americans are getting has dropped by an average of 1.5–2 hours per day. Studies show that people are more inclined to snack on junk foods when they are sleep-deprived. In fact, when people were asked to explain why they engaged in snacking, one of the main reasons cited was "to gain energy." A lack of sleep plays havoc with the hormones, ghrelin and leptin, which control appetite and satiety. Satiety is the feeling of being full after eating, which may become impaired when you are tired. A frequent urge to snack may indicate that you need more sleep rather than more food.

More than two-thirds of Americans are currently overweight or obese. An *epidemic* is a disease that spreads rapidly among many people at the same time and the rising tide of obesity has been called not just an epidemic, but a tsunami. Obesity is increasing the risk for diabetes, gallstones, osteoarthritis, breast and colon cancer, heart attack, stroke and other diseases. Moreover, Americans are not alone. Obesity is spreading around the globe and the ramifications are startling. A 2014 McKinsey Report states that obesity costs the global economy approximately $2 trillion a year in health-related absences and costs.

It is mind-boggling to contemplate the number of calories in meals that most people consider "normal." Fast foods loaded with calories, such as cheeseburgers or pizza, are often eaten at lunch or dinner. Portion sizes have increased over time and the average fast food or restaurant meal now contains 1000-1500 calories. Unless we are digging ditches all day or running marathons, this is far more than any of us needs at a single meal.

Research has shown that the more often people eat fast food, the greater their chances of gaining weight. The amount of food we eat *increases* as the effort to obtain it *decreases*. At my maximum weight, and after a stressful day at work, I remember frequent drive-through orders that were tasty and inexpensive. Now I know that I didn't need those empty calories for energy, which is why they were being stored as fat. There's a simple formula that I recall whenever I get the urge to head for a drive-through:

Excess calories = BODY FAT

And what effect do the super-sized and larger portion sizes have on most people and on calorie intake? People served larger portions eat more food than those served smaller portions, regardless of the food item. For example, people at a restaurant who were served 50% more pasta ate 43% more than people served the normal portion size.

These and many other studies documenting the effect of portion size have been published by Dr. Brian Wansink, author of *Mindless Eating: Why We Eat More Than We Think*. Wansink and colleagues have demonstrated that people consume more than 90% of the food on their plate *even if they are not hungry*. Participants in the studies refused to believe they were affected by portion size, even when they were shown the data.

The response to portion size is a result of our automatic habits and brain responses to large quantities of tasty food whether they are served in a restaurant or at home. This is a facet of human behavior that applies to all of us regardless of our weight.

Because super-sized servings are so common, we have become accustomed to thinking that big meals are normal and that we need to eat a lot of food to feel satisfied. The truth is that our bodies don't need anywhere near that much food. Wansink's studies have shown that smaller portions can satisfy our hunger and cravings just as well as larger portions. In one remarkable study, people fed large portions of food, containing 1370 calories, ate 77% more food than people given much smaller portions of food containing only 195 calories. However, within fifteen minutes of the meal, participants who ate the smaller portion were just as satisfied as those who ate the large portion.

There are all kinds of ways to use this knowledge to lose weight. First, check out the calorie counts of the meals at your favorite restaurant so you know what you are consuming before you order. Many restaurants have meal calorie counts posted online, so you can identify and avoid the highest-calorie entrees before you go. Second, you can split a restaurant entree with a friend, or simply divide your restaurant meal in half before you start. If you take the uneaten half home, you can get two meals for the price of one. One caveat: you need to resolve in advance to cut the meal in half or your automatic reflex will be to eat the whole meal.

High-sugar/high-fat foods → overeating

It's not only large portions that cause overeating. It is the very nature of highly processed foods, which are designed to be hyperpalatable. Do you remember the potato chip campaign that taunted us with the slogan,

"Betcha can't eat just one"? It turns out they were right. Potato chip consumption in the U.S. went from 11.4 pounds per person in 1960 to 19.3 pounds per person in 2007. A long-term study showed that potato chip consumption is a significant contributor to overeating and weight gain.

We'd like to think that we can eat just a few chips, but studies show otherwise. Individuals given large bags of potato chips tripled the amount of chips they ate compared with individuals given small bags. Amazingly, the people who ate the large portions usually *did not believe* they had eaten more than people given normal-sized portions. In addition, both groups felt equally full, whether they had eaten the smaller or larger portion. It is a scientific truth that in most eating situations, eating is an automatic response to temptations, cues, and portion sizes.

To shed light on the power of the potato chip, Dr. Tobias Hoch from the University of Erlangen-Nuremberg studied animals that had a choice of standard chow or chow with added potato chips. When potato chips were added to a chow diet, the animals ate more food. Dr. Hoch and colleagues showed that the combination of fat and carbohydrates in snack foods can trigger *hedonic hyperphagia*: eating for pleasure rather than for need. In short, potato chips stimulate the reward center in the brain – the same area that is involved in the development of drug addictions.

Foods that are high in fat, sugar, and salt stimulate the appetite so that we may eat more than we need. Dr. Ashley Gearhardt states, "The food environment has changed dramatically with the influx of hyperpalatable foods that are engineered in ways that appear to surpass the rewarding properties of traditional foods – such as vegetables, fruits, and nuts - by increasing fat, sugar, salt, flavors, and food additives to high levels."

And speaking of engineered "foods," consider the chemical composition of corn chips and potato chips. Although the manufacturing process starts with corn or potatoes, the final product is highly processed. One popular brand of tortilla chips contains 34 different ingredients including oil, salt, sugar, MSG, malic acid, sodium acetate, disodium inosate, disodium guanylate, citric acid, artificial flavors, and maltodextrin. Maltodextrin is a form of carbohydrate with a high glycemic index, meaning that it causes a spike in blood sugar. The glycemic index of foods is important because there is a known link between blood glucose levels and the activation of brain regions that are involved with addiction. MSG is a flavor enhancer that has been associated with weight gain through mechanisms that are being investigated.

The bottom line is that if highly processed foods are around the house, we are highly likely to eat them in addition to our regular meals. It's no wonder that Americans' weights are skyrocketing.

You might think that eating occurs because internal hunger mechanisms automatically trigger eating. In the modern environment, this is rarely the case. Instead, eating is often an automatic reaction to the environment. If we are unaware that eating is an automatic behavior, we may not be able to avoid acting on what we perceive as a real need. We simply respond, and wonder why we continue to gain weight.

Hyperpalatable foods provoke a subconscious desire to eat regardless of a need for calories. Sugar is the main culprit and when sugar is combined with fat, the effects are magnified. The problem with sugar is not just that it produces obesity. Sugar consumption also has been linked to increased rates of Type 2 diabetes and cardiovascular disease.

Between 1950 and 2005, the consumption of added sugars increased by a whopping 43 pounds per person per year. The average American consumes approximately 300 calories per day from added sugar, and the top 20% of sugar consumers take in more than *700 calories per day* from added sugar. Perhaps we should call that trend *the icing on the cake*. The World Health Organization recommends limiting added sugars to no more than 10% of total calories. Nearly 60% of the population exceeds the recommended limit.

The main sources of added sugar are soft drinks, fruit drinks, grain-based desserts such as cookies, cakes, brownies and pies, and dairy desserts such as ice cream. These foods are loaded with empty calories. And for women who binge, the foods that are cited as being craved are those with high amounts of sugar combined with fat: chocolate, candy, cookies, brownies, ice cream, and cakes. In these foods, over 90% of the calories are contributed by sugar and fat. In the next chapter, we'll examine the effects of hyperpalatable foods on the brain and overeating.

IMPLEMENTATION

Hyperpalatable foods provoke a desire to eat at the subconscious level regardless of a need for calories. Sugar is the main culprit and when sugar is combined with fat, the effects are magnified.

1. How much sugar are you consuming? List the top five sources of sugar in your diet and how often / how much you consume.
2. Are you willing to free yourself from the effects of sugar? Write down any concerns you may have, and consider possible solutions.

wine
ice cream

4

Why We Overeat

We can alter the chemistry
provided we have the courage to dissect the elements.
~ ANAÏS NIN

By the time we're adults, we have developed billions of neural pathways by modeling others, experimenting on our own, and even visualizing the future. These comfortable circuits regulate our behavior. Unfortunately, many overeaters have nonproductive, automatic, and unhealthy eating patterns. The good news is that we can use our logical pre-frontal cortex to practice new thoughts and behaviors, inhibit our pre-programmed impulses, and ultimately rewire circuits. Effective weight-loss involves delaying, changing, and shifting automatic behaviors as well as planning and implementing new eating and activity choices.

At a basic level, it's important to know how our brains work in order to understand our eating and overeating. Let's take a very simplistic look at two brain systems that control eating.

First, there is the homeostatic system, centered in the hypothalamus, which is designed to maintain a balance between calories expended and calories consumed. Many diet books focus on this system because eating when you are hungry and stopping when you are full is a pretty solid concept.

Second, there is the non-homeostatic system, which is related to the brain's reward circuitry. The reward system enables our brains to take special notice of experiences such as eating and sex. The term "reward-driven eating" refers to eating that is driven by sensory pleasure and by the sight or smell of hyper-palatable foods. These foods often motivate us to eat right now, or over-eat at a meal, even if one intended to abstain or to eat moderately. Therefore, reward-driven eating is a strong contributor to weight gain and obesity.

The motivational component of food reward is largely mediated by the mesolimbic dopamine system, which also mediates the motivation to engage in sex, gambling, and substance use. The ventral tegmental area (VTA) and nucleus accumbens are key components of reward pathways. See the diagram below.

BRAIN REWARD PATHWAYS

Scientists have discovered regions within the brain that are stimulated by all types of reinforcing stimuli including food and many drugs of abuse

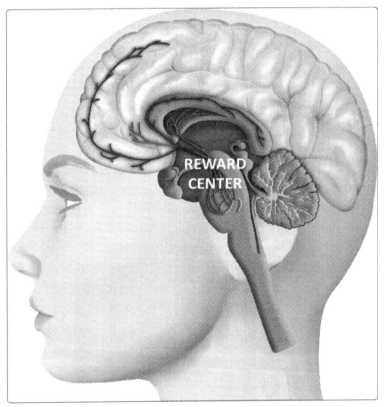

Image via Wikimedia Commons |Public Domain| by Arias-Carrión, Oscar, et al. from: International Archives of Medicine 7.1 (2014): 29.

When pleasurable eating occurs there is a release of dopamine in the reward center of the brain. The dopamine response motivates us to repeat the food-seeking or drug-seeking behavior.

The stimulating effects of food or drugs on the reward center can be visualized with functional magnetic resonance imaging (fMRI) scans of the brain. When hyperpalatable foods are consumed, oxygen-rich arterial blood flows into the activated area and displaces oxygen-poor venous blood. When viewed with fMRI, it looks as if the brain is lit up in that area. "The more desirable something is, the more significant the changes in blood flow in that part of the brain," states Harvard University's Dr. Uma Karmarkar.

The reward system lies within the emotionally "hot" system described by Drs. Walter Mischel and Janet Metcalfe from Columbia University. The "hot" system is linked to desire: it wants what it wants, and it wants it *now*. It is not even necessary to consume the food to activate the reward center; merely *seeing an image of hyperpalatable food* will do the trick. As a result, such images serve as cues that can trigger overeating of hyperpalatable foods.

When faced with a strong temptation, the reward system goes into overdrive and motivates us to acquire and consume the tempting food. And in our obesogenic environment, the average person is faced with over 200 food decisions every single day. That's more than a dozen decisions every waking hour, on average. It's no wonder that, in many cases, people succumb to the temptation to eat. In a study of human participants, the mere sight of chocolate increased consumption *even when individuals were highly satiated.*

With hyperpalatable foods such as chocolate, ice cream or cookies, the combination of sugar and fat is particularly potent. The dietary fat causes the release of opioids in the brain, and the opioids potentiate the effects of sugar. Therefore, high-sugar/high-fat foods trigger desire and make us want to repeat the experience. Routine overeating of ice cream, cookies and the like can lead to adaptations in the reward center of the brain, so that more and more dopamine or opioid is needed to get the same effect, creating dependence.

Dr. Kelly Brownell, an internationally renowned expert on obesity, says, "Everybody knows that some food products are intensely palatable or habit forming. Just like drugs of abuse, brain-rewarding effects or reinforcement from food products can lead to loss of control." Studies of animals have shown that the loss of control is rooted in biology. When animals are allowed to choose between sugar and intravenous cocaine, they overwhelmingly choose sugar.

Compulsive overeaters and drug abusers experience *cravings*. A craving can be something we are aware of - a conscious state of desire - or a subconscious motivation to obtain the object of desire. Since brain responses associated with cravings can be visualized with MRI, it may not surprise you to learn that the food industry is investing in *neuromarketing*. Neuromarketing involves studying subconscious brain activity to find out what really makes human brains "light up." As an article in Fast Company says, "These corporations share the same goal: to mine your brain so they can blow your mind with products you deeply desire."

Once a subconscious script (high-sugar/high-fat food = stimulation and positive feeling) becomes imprinted in the brain, the behavior it dictates becomes so automatic that we respond before we're even conscious of a stimulus. Even a *memory* of a rewarding event can stimulate the release of dopamine and cause cravings for the object of desire. The overconsumption of rewarding substances becomes habitual, unintentional, and involuntary. In fact, habits can be defined as:

Learned sequences of acts
that have been *reinforced* in the past *by rewarding experiences,*
and that are *triggered by the environment* to produce behavior,
largely *outside* of people's conscious awareness.

Under the influence of habits, the brain makes decisions instantaneously and automatically. A way to think about eating and other automatic behaviors is that it is like being on autopilot. Autopilot mode is a good thing if the plane is on the right course, but a bad thing if the weather has blown the plane off course. When we overeat and are blown off course, we need our conscious, analytical mind – our Captain, if you will - to intervene and get the plane back on course. Our Captain is capable of taking executive action unless he/she is unaware that the plane is headed off course. We can't expect to override our automatic responses until we are aware of them. So, in the face of strong habits, we tend to do whatever we have done in the past.

To sum up, our obesogenic environment can trigger overeating at the subconscious level with an effect that is largely outside of our conscious awareness. The good news is that we can become attuned to the daily cues in our own lives and develop proactive plans – including implementation intentions - to interrupt our automatic reflexes. To formulate a personal plan for temptations and cravings, become fully aware of the external cues for overeating and how they undermine our intentions to lose weight.

IMPLEMENTATION

Food intake is regulated by two basic drives. One drive involves the homeo-static system, which is designed to meet our energy needs. It operates through sensations of hunger and satiety. The other drive is the non-homeostatic (reward-driven) system which can trigger eating regardless of hunger.

A regular meal schedule (about every four hours), including some protein and fiber at each meal, helps to provide satiety. Reward-driven eating can be prevented by avoiding hyperpalatable foods and food cues.

1. In your daily/weekly life, how many eating episodes are driven by hunger versus reward?
2. If you ate when you were not hungry, what triggered the eating episode?
3. What is your overall eating pattern? How are your calories allocated between meals and snacks? Are you eating three meals a day or grazing all day long?
4. Do you know what hunger and satiety "feel" like? Use the *Am I Hungry?* Table to assess your hunger.

AM I HUNGRY?	
When you eat, you want to be hungry, not starving. Get in touch with your hunger by rating yourself before and 20 minutes after eating an adequate amount of food. Here's a numerical rating you can use to assess whether you're hungry.	
5	Starving
4	Stomach growling
3	Mildly hungry (last ate over 2 hours ago.) Maybe a glass of water, waiting 20 minutes, or eating a piece of fruit will tide me over until mealtime.
2	Satisfied but am thinking about additional food
1	Ate too much, uncomfortable

5

The Role of Cues in Overeating

To learn new habits is everything,
for it is to reach the substance of life.
Life is but a tissue of habits.
~ HENRI FREDERIC AMIEL

As a habitual behavior, eating is predominantly <u>in</u>voluntary and <u>un</u>intentional, and it is guided by situational cues. Eye-tracking technology confirms that people's eyes often are riveted to high-sugar foods, even though they are not aware of the effect. We are bombarded with temptations, and like it or not, we often respond.

High-sugar/high-fat foods are available not only at the supermarket but at gas stations, office supply stores, hardware stores, big box stores – in short, everywhere. Candy and soft drinks that are loaded with sugar are placed at checkout stands so we will have plenty of time to look at them while we are standing in line. This is a successful marketing strategy because these displays trigger impulse purchases.

More than half of all food purchasing decisions are unplanned. An important determinant of purchasing is how much an item attracts our attention; this is known as *salience*. Salience is the state or quality by which an object stands out relative to its neighbors. Large product displays are more salient than smaller displays. When the amount of shelf space for a consumer item is doubled in grocery stores, sales of that item increase by about 40%. Hyperpalatable foods, which stimulate the reward system, have the additional property known as *incentive salience*. In other words, they provoke *wanting*. Hyperpalatable foods produce a desire for more high-sugar/high-fat foods as demonstrated in the following formula.

**Hyperpalatable foods → reward system →
↑ desire for hyperpalatable foods**

Because of the strong link between candy displays, impulse purchases and obesity, the Center for Science in the Public Interest (CSPI) recommends that non-food stores stop selling foods and beverages at checkout stands. Unless and until that happens, people who want to avoid impulse purchases will need to develop their own strategies and tactics to counteract the temptations.

One proactive strategy is to establish implementation intentions, also known as if-then plans, for temptations you encounter in your daily life. Here is an example of an implementation intention: "If I am at the checkout stand, I will turn my back to the candy display, focus my attention on my purchases, and remind myself that sweets are not a good choice for me. I will stick to my grocery list – no impulse purchases." Implementation intentions are effective tools for habit change that involve being aware of the cues in your own life so you can be proactive.

Cues often come in the form of commercials that display juicy, sizzling foods with people opening their mouths to take a big bite. These cues trigger brain and hormone responses and cause us to experience the desire to eat even when we are not hungry. This is known as *priming*. Researchers from Yale University observed that adults and children who watched a TV show with food commercials ate significantly more snack food than those who watched the same show with non-food commercials. Cooking shows have the same effect.

The increased snacking and cravings that occur in response to commercials are a result of unconscious mental processes. In the Yale study, most participants did not recognize the influence of food advertising on their eating behaviors. These unconscious processes explain why will-power often fails when it comes to temptations. The neurons that signal the presence of a reward are already firing, and motivating us to act, before we are aware of the cue. Trying to suppress the impulse is like closing the barn door after the horse has bolted. A far better strategy is to mute the food commercials as soon as they appear.

Advertisers know that shoppers often purchase snacks through simple reminders of how tired, hungry, or thirsty they are. Hunger and thirst are "hot-states" that reduce immediate self-control. Thus nutritionists advise people not to shop for food when they are hungry, because hungry people are more likely to succumb to salient displays. The compulsion to act on these "hot" impulses is called *hot-state decision making*. For reasons of physiology and brain chemistry, if we are overweight we are more susceptible to food cues. Hot-state cues can be avoided by steering clear of the display, with the help of implementation intentions. Implementation intentions have successfully been used to help people stop smoking and eliminate other addictive behaviors.

In addition to showing people guzzling high-calorie foods, commercials associate such foods with fun and happiness. If you step back and analyze commercial messages, you'll see that the promise of happiness is everywhere. The reason for this is simple: the promise of happiness boosts sales. A "happy" brand is a successful brand: it is better liked and chosen more often. As writer Ross Klein observed in *Marketing Happiness in an Unhappy World*, "Successful marketers understand and respond to the human condition... surreptitiously, worming their way into the corner of the consumer's mind where fear resides, they offer solace with a promise of happiness after consumption." Ads that urge us to "unleash spontaneous moments of joy" and "discover our personal euphoria" are everywhere.

If we believe the advertisements, we may buy into the myth that chocolate, ice cream, all-you-can-eat buffets, and greasy foods deliver fun, joy, happiness, euphoria, and friends. I used to think that hyperpalatable foods were rewards, but not anymore. These advertisements are peddling a fantasy. Ads never show the reality of food cravings, compulsions, weight gain, or out-of-control eating. Instead they feature happy, energetic, attractive people who are perpetually thin despite consuming unhealthy foods. It has been shown that the use of thin ideal models prompts people who are trying to cut back to eat *more* chocolate, not less.

Much as with any substance that can be abused, chocolate and other hyperpalatable foods are associated with cravings. In one study when cravers viewed pictures of chocolate, the images activated regions of the brain known to be involved in habit-forming behaviors and drug addiction. As you begin to take note of your own cravings, strive to identify the cue that triggered the craving.

Food companies and restaurants capitalize on the power of slogans to remind us of our cravings, luring us with adjectives such as "irresistible," "craveable," "rewards," and – all subtlety aside – "addictive." We recently saw a food review with the headline, "This cheesecake should come with a warning label – *ADDICTIVE*." And then there is the word *chocoholic* as in "Here's to the *chocoholics*." A *chocoholic* is a person who craves or compulsively consumes chocolate.

Commercials that remind us of our cravings can motivate us subconsciously to take action to satisfy them. We're not even aware that we are being manipulated by the cue. Reminders of cravings are presumed to be harmless, even cute, because people have free will – at least in theory. But the obesity epidemic suggests that cravings are not harmless.

The consumption and overconsumption of high-sugar/high-fat foods create an expectation of pleasure that pulls us in. Unfortunately the promise is a false one. The "moment of joy" that comes from consuming a chocolate bar or a carton of ice cream is – quite literally –momentary. A few minutes later, the joy is gone. We consume more and more, hoping for the joy that we were promised. It begins to sound like a compulsion. For this reason, Dr. Robert Lustig, the author of *Sugar – The Bitter Truth*, calls sugar "the most unhappy of pleasures." Just as philosophers have known for centuries, happiness does *not* lie in consumption, whether it is a soft drink, candy bar, or a carton of ice cream.

Temptations arise frequently and they act on the reward system of the brain. When dealing with temptations, many dieters try to exert willpower, with limited success – and we now know why. Many studies have shown that even the strongest willpower can be eroded by constant exposure to high-sugar/high-fat foods, distractions, sleeplessness, and stress.

For me, one of the best strategies was to avoid high-sugar/high-fat temptations altogether, by getting them all out of the house *and replacing them* with satisfying, tasty, nutrient-dense foods. I eliminated all sugar products from my home and assigned a negative label to junk foods that did nothing to fuel my energy. In essence, I was relabeling and avoiding former "reward foods" that made me larger and less healthy while I established new habits consistent with my goals.

My strategy of proactive avoidance is supported by numerous studies showing that we are more likely to succeed if we avoid hyperpalatable foods *before* they trigger an automatic impulse to consume. The 13th century adage "Out of sight, out of mind" is as true today as it was over 800 years ago. Just as smokers are more likely to quit if they get cigarettes and ashtrays out of the house, compulsive eaters are more likely to regain control if they eliminate hyperpalatable foods from the home.

Dr. Jeffrey Quinn at Duke University reports that study participants who were trying to resist temptations were able to inhibit their strong impulses by removing themselves from the tempting stimulus. Dr. Molly Crockett at the University of Oxford says, "Our research suggests that the most effective way to beat temptations is to avoid facing them in the first place." And Dr. Sherry Pagoto at the University of Massachusetts says that "[Refined] foods need to be completely eliminated so that they stop hijacking your brain, giving you a chance to regain control."

When hyperpalatable foods are removed from your immediate environment, the automatic links between cues and habits are disrupted, giving your conscious mind a chance to recall your weight-loss intentions. Then, in deciding whether or not to fulfill a craving, your mind will factor in the effort of making a trip out to purchase something you really don't need. After considering the costs and rewards of your actions, you still might decide to expend the effort, but at least it will be a conscious decision rather than an automatic one. The distinction is an important one.

The good news is that new, healthy habits can become *just as automatic as unhealthy habits* by surrounding ourselves with healthy foods and by practicing healthy eating, one day at a time until new subconscious scripts and habits are formed. Imagine the process of change as a journey, much like traveling abroad and trying out new foods. It's a journey worth taking.

IMPLEMENTATION

Control Your Environment is the third scientific principle of weight-loss success. More than half of all food purchasing decisions are impulsive (unplanned) and many purchases are triggered by retail displays. Television, billboards, electronic and print media also influence our desire and subsequent purchase of advertised foods. Once hyperpalatable foods are in the home, they are impossible to avoid.

1. What will you do to eliminate high-sugar/high-fat foods from your home?
2. When you see a commercial for a food or a restaurant, analyze the ad. How is the promise of happiness incorporated into the ad?
3. Reframe the way you think about the promise. What are some things you would say to the food manufacturer or advertiser?
4. The next time you are watching television, try hitting the 'mute' button whenever a food commercial starts. Formulate this as an implementation intention (*If a food commercial comes on the television, I will hit the 'mute' button.*)
5. Does the absence of sound change your perception of the food?
6. Name five other frequently-encountered food cues in your life. What will you do when cues and triggers occur? Using the following *Implementation Intentions* table as a model, create your own strategies for dealing with cues and triggers.

IMPLEMENTATION INTENTIONS	
Here are some examples of implementation intentions. Using this table as a guide, formulate your own intentions for situations you encounter in your daily life.	
SITUATION	**IMPLEMENTATION INTENTION**
Candy at the checkout stand	If I am at the checkout stand, I will turn my back to the candy display, focus my attention on my purchases, and remind myself that sugar is not a good choice for me.
Supermarket	If I go to the supermarket, I will stick to the perimeter of the store where the fresh foods are located. I will stick to my grocery list and avoid the chips, candy and soft drink aisles.
Potluck or buffet	If I am going to a potluck or buffet, I will fill up my plate with salad, vegetables and fruit instead of eating everything in sight. I will not go hungry.
Restaurant	If I am going to a restaurant, I will suggest sharing an entrée with a friend, or I will eat half the entrée and ask for a box.
Restaurant	If the waiter offers bread or chips I'll say "no thanks." I'll drink a glass of water before the meal. If the waiter offers dessert, I will say "I'll just have coffee."
Birthday party	If I'm going to a birthday party, I'll remember that my happiest celebrations were a result of connections with people and healthy foods. I'll make sure to focus on others and fill up on the nutrient-dense foods.
Game Day party	If I am invited to a game day party, I will offer to bring raw veggies and low-calorie dip.
Cravings	If I have a craving for chocolate or ice cream, I will set a timer for 20 minutes. I will go for a walk or do something else until the craving subsides.
Negative emotions	If I'm overwhelmed by negative emotions, I'll write in my journal, visualize what I want to achieve through weight-loss and maintenance, and eat some vegetable soup if I'm really hungry.

6

Eat Mindfully

*It's a transformative experience to simply pause
instead of immediately filling up the space.
By waiting, we begin to connect with fundamental restlessness
as well as fundamental spaciousness.*
~ PEMA CHÖDRÖN, FROM *WHEN THINGS FALL APART*

I know now that I was not always present or mindful when I ate. When I was stressed, tired, and trying to do too many things at once, I'd forget about my intentions to lose weight and just reach for the M&Ms. Studies confirm that we are more likely to eat mindlessly when we are occupied with multiple tasks or other problems. I knew that I had to break the cycle of automatic, habitual behaviors by incorporating specific strategies so that I would be cognizant of what, when, and why I ate. In essence, I was determined to make the unconscious conscious. The mindset that made this possible for me is known as *mindfulness*.

Dr. Ellen Langer of Harvard University, who pioneered the psychological concept of mindfulness, points out that many times others can detect our mindlessness (*The lights are on but nobody is home*) even before we do. As Dr. Langer said in an interview on National Public Radio, "No one gains 10 pounds overnight." Her advice? Mindfulness or simple noticing.

The various facets of mindfulness are rooted in Buddhism, an Eastern religion practiced by over 300 million people around the world. While the Buddhist practice has been around for over 2,500 years, the practice and attitude of mindfulness has just taken hold in the United States in the last forty years. According to Dr. Jon Kabat-Zinn, author of *Wherever*

You Go, There You Are, mindfulness is the awareness that arises through paying attention in a particular way: on purpose, in the present moment, and nonjudgmentally. It is defined as bringing one's complete attention to the experiences occurring *in the present moment* in a nonjudgmental and non-reactive way. Mindfulness training is being used in many treatment programs for smoking, binge eating, and drug abuse.

The five facets of mindfulness are observing, describing, acting with awareness, non-judging of inner experience, and non-reactivity to inner experience. Each stage of mindfulness has special meaning for me. *Observing* means attending to or noticing internal and external stimuli, such as sensations, emotions, cognitions, sights, sounds, and smells, without reacting. In order to develop this skill, I take walks in nature, visually exploring as if I were seeing the beauty around me for the first time. The important part of observing is, as Professor Richard Alpert (popularly known as Ram Dass) once said, "Be Here Now."

Describing, which refers to labeling experiences with words, has the effect of reducing our emotional reactivity to experiences. Writing in a journal helped me to develop *noticing without reacting* by disrupting automatic reactions to cravings. If I got the urge to go out for a Big Mac or some chocolate, I would set a timer for twenty minutes, write in my journal, drink a glass of home-made sugar-free lemonade or pursue another activity. I basically intervened in my potentially automatic behavior and established a new set of habits.

I practice *acting with awareness* every time I plan, prepare, and eat a meal. I am mindful of what and why I'm eating so that I can experience joy and appreciation of food that empowers my mind and body.

When I'm mindful, I'm aware of my judgments and reactions. I've found that negative judgments and reactions are primarily based on past experiences or in worries about the future. When I focus on the here and now, I am able to more clearly see what is actually happening in my life. There's an inner calm that facilitates a healthy lifestyle.

Since eating is an automatic behavior that often occurs mindlessly, it's not surprising that we can prevent automatic snacking if we become aware of the cues. When we behave mindfully, we pause for a moment and become fully aware of what is going on, both externally (sights, sounds, and smells) and internally (sensations, emotions, and thoughts). In essence, we are substituting alternative behaviors - *noticing, describing*, and *nonjudgment* - before we reach for the M&Ms.

MINDFULNESS: 5 STEPS

Observing

Describing

Acting with Awareness

Non-judging of Inner Experience

Non-reactivity to Inner Experience

In order to make the unconscious conscious, I kept a detailed journal, writing down everything I ate as well as my physical activity every day. My journaling enabled me to uncover the habit loop associated with my overeating. Through mindful journaling, I discovered the following pattern:

First, I would experience a *trigger*. A trigger is anything such as an act or event that serves as a stimulus and initiates a reaction or series of reactions. Two of my common internal triggers focused on having a lot of work to do in a short period of time and dealing with conflict.

Second, my subconscious or, in some instances, conscious reaction to the trigger would be that I needed a simple way to cope with a difficult situation or emotion.

Third, I coped by eating high-sugar/high-fat foods (my former reward).

Fourth, eating hyperpalatable foods kept the habit entrenched. The effect of sugar and fat on my brain was powerful and continued to reinforce overeating.

Once I identified this automatic habit loop, I knew that I could either remove the stressor or use stress reduction to break the cycle. One of the most successful tools that I employed was to slow down, become truly aware of what I was thinking and feeling, and wait at least twenty minutes before I ate anything. My favorite and most successful substitute behavior was to exercise. Instead of grabbing food, take a walk after a stressful day.

Keeping a journal, getting in touch with how I felt, and identifying triggers, facilitated my weight loss as I found replacements for automatic eating. Now, when I work at my computer, I take a brief exercise break every 45 minutes and I've eliminated eating and working at the same time.

Mindfulness is a powerful tool for getting in touch with your behaviors so that you can substitute a healthy and positive response for an automatic reaction.

What a liberation
to realize that the 'voice in my head' is not who I am.
'Who am I, then?'
The one who sees that.
~ ECKHART TOLLE

TACKLING EMOTIONAL EATING

Rumination, absorption in the past, or anxieties about the future can pull one away from the present and facilitate mindless eating. Periods of stress or negative mood are often associated with the consumption of hyper-palatable foods, giving rise to the terms "comfort foods" and "emotional eating." Emotional eating is a major reason why many weight loss plans fail. If you can find ways to prevent or interrupt the impulses that cause emotional eating, you are more likely to succeed.

In psychology, a tactic known as *cognitive defusion* is an effective way of dealing with negative emotions so that they do not automatically trigger overeating or other unhealthy behaviors. Cognitive defusion is a form of metacognition or *thinking about what you are thinking* in order to change your thinking.

The idea behind cognitive defusion is that when we are overly engaged or "fused" with our thoughts, the thoughts are automatically presumed to be legitimate and demanding of immediate action. In contrast, when we take the perspective of an observer of our own thoughts, we are more able to experience negative feelings without instinctively responding to them. As psychologist Dr. Lucie Hemmen explains, "Such people experience emotions richly but cultivate an ability to stay calm, composed and effective in the face of them. They experience a pleasant shift in power, feeling more as though they are having their emotions than their emotions are 'having' them."

Even cravings that seem to dominate our attention will fade away if we distract ourselves by doing something else, focus on the future consequences instead of the immediate temptation, or detach from our cravings by viewing them as transient impulses that will fade away. To illustrate the point, researchers studied participants who were trying to cut back on their chocolate consumption. The participants who were taught to "step back" from their cravings ate significantly less chocolate than the control group in the study.

At its core, mindfulness entails an attitude of curiosity about life and our own experiences, perceptions, and behaviors. For me, mindfulness is living in the moment, being aware of how I feel, being clear about my long-term goals, identifying emotional triggers that can sabotage my health, and self-monitoring what, when, and why I eat. As you practice mindful awareness and non-reactivity you gradually lose your fear of out-of-control eating because you begin to recognize the triggers and develop alternative coping strategies.

Mindfulness has a ripple effect that will help you with other life issues. Most people would agree that a lot of our unhappiness comes from the mind's constant chatter as it jumps from one life-worry, conflict, or stressful event to another. A Harvard study confirmed that there's a clear connection between mind-wandering and unhappiness. Mindfulness improves the ability to focus one's thoughts on the task at hand instead of ruminating or getting caught up in a "monkey mind" of unhappy or stress-inducing thoughts. As a trait, mindfulness has been associated with a lower frequency of negative automatic thoughts and with an enhanced ability to relinquish, rather than obsessing about, those thoughts.

The practice of mindfulness has profound long-term benefits. I can honestly say that since I've become more mindful, previously difficult or tedious tasks such as budgeting, cleaning, and even chopping vegetables have become more pleasurable. In short, mindfulness improves our ability to shift from unhealthy to healthy patterns of thought and behavior.

IMPLEMENTATION

Eat Mindfully is the fourth scientific principle of weight-loss success. Evaluate your behaviors to identify your habit loops and identify, reframe, and redirect nonproductive behaviors and thinking. Use the following *Habit Loop for Overeating* table to help you to explain your habit loops.

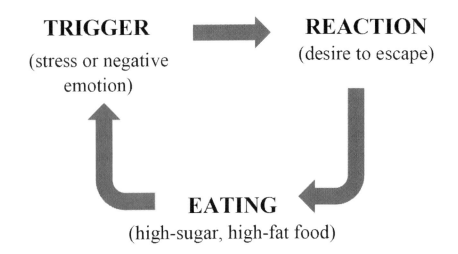

TRIGGER
(stress or negative emotion)

REACTION
(desire to escape)

EATING
(high-sugar, high-fat food)

	HABIT LOOP FOR OVEREATING
	Through journaling and mindful awareness, I discovered the following habit loop:
1	I would experience a negative trigger. A trigger is any act or event that serves as a stimulus and initiates a reaction or series of reactions. Two of my common internal triggers focused on having a lot of work to do in a relatively short period of time, and dealing with conflict.
2	My subconscious or, in some instances, conscious reaction to the trigger would be that I needed a simple way to cope with this difficult situation or to escape from unproductive emotions.
3	I coped by eating high-sugar/high-fat foods (my former reward).
4	Eating hyperpalatable foods kept the habit entrenched. The effect of sugar on my brain was powerful and continued to reinforce overeating.

7

Visualize Your Goal

A vision is not just a picture of what could be;
it is an appeal to our better selves,
a call to become something more.
~ ROSABETH MOSS KANTER

I f you can visualize what you want to accomplish, you can achieve it. Today, sports psychologists, Olympic and professional athletes, politicians, entrepreneurs, and folks like us who want to achieve our goals are testimony to the power of visualization. In fact, visualization is an excellent tool to help you to achieve and maintain your weight goal.

Visualization is a cognitive tool that enables humans to form a mental picture of a future situation, interaction, or success as if it were a current reality. According to practitioners of visualization, the process can increase motivation and concentration as well as reduce fear and anxiety. Many people have used both attitudinal and behavioral visualization to assist with weight loss and other life goals.

Visualization =
Increased Motivation and Concentration

The power of visualization lies in the fact that before we can achieve a future goal, we must have a realistic idea of what it will look like and how we will achieve it.

Visualize this thing that you want,
See it, feel it, believe in it.
Make your mental blue print, and begin to build.
~ ROBERT COLLIER

Throughout my weight loss and maintenance, I used visualization to create mental films of a thinner me. When I began my weight loss journey, I owned a favorite sweater and skirt that I had outgrown. Due to weight gain, I could not button the sweater or zip the skirt. So, I visualized myself wearing the clothes with great confidence and contentment. Another mental film was a 5K race in which I would participate and enjoy. My 5K film became so detailed that I could view the race from both a subjective point of view as if I were running in the race and an objective perspective as if I were an observer in the audience. A third mental film focused on preparing and presenting a lovely nutrient-dense holiday meal with pride, confidence, and comfort to a group of family and friends.

What I found is that it's important to visualize the "major final film" as well as smaller episodes. While one of my big films was participating in a 5K race, smaller episodes that contributed to my final success included hiking a nature trail, cooking nutrient-dense foods, and participating in a yoga class to increase flexibility. The point is to be realistic about your visualizations and include smaller mental films that will help you to visualize and accomplish the steps that lead to a big success.

When I first started my program, I visualized my mental films every day and then after about four months when my behaviors became more engrained and I was actualizing my goal, I viewed them less often. Make visualizations as clear, vivid, and detailed as possible so that you can see, feel, and experience what it would be like to exercise easier, wear smaller sizes, and feel better. Recently I wore the sweater (the skirt is too large now) and felt confident and content as I realized that my mental films were now realities.

Another visualization technique involved contrasting heavier images of me with ones at my goal weight. Studies have confirmed that being aware of the discrepancy between the present and the future can promote behaviors to move towards the goal.

In a study of people who wanted to lose weight, participants were asked to visualize their weight problem solved. This is the equivalent of me visualizing my "thin" photos. Then the participants were asked to think about the negative aspects of reality – the fact that the types of foods they were eating were keeping them overweight. With both images in mind, participants were asked to compare their goal with reality of their present situation. Participants who adopted this approach were the most successful in their weight loss efforts.

A recent study confirms that my approach of vividly imagining the future boosts weight loss. Volunteers who were overweight were asked to "bring the future to life" by vividly imagining themselves being present at a joyous event at a future point in time. After the visualization exercise, they were shown plates of cookies, French fries, and other tempting foods, and asked to rate their appeal. They were then told to eat as much of the food as they liked. Those who had visualized themselves in the future, as if it were happening *today*, consumed far fewer calories than the control group in the study.

In an online post, Wray Herbert, the author of *On Second Thought: Outsmarting your Mind's Hard-Wired Habits*, says: "It's possible that being in the future – through imagery – somehow improves the ability to perceive the real value of delaying rewards. That is, we may know the value in the abstract, but it's tough to make real-life decisions based on abstractions. When we actually put ourselves into the future, we're experiencing the consequences of our decisions rather than merely calculating them."

Visualizing the future as if we were living it right now – seeing ourselves actually wearing the clothes we want to wear, looking healthy and attractive in a slimmer body - helps us focus on the longer-term reward. You begin to associate the old way of eating with being overweight and uncomfortable, and the new way of eating with being slimmer and feeling great.

My most successful mental films were ones that resulted in great visceral feelings that outweighed cravings or other emotions that could lead to overeating. Wearing my smaller size sweater in my mental film was motivating. Wearing the sweater now is exciting. The author William Clement Stone spoke the truth when he stated, "Whatever the mind can conceive, it can achieve."

IMPLEMENTATION

Visualize Your Future is the fifth scientific principle of weight-loss success. We're with Walt Disney on this one: "If you can dream it, you can do it."

What inspires you to eat well and exercise? Think about what you want to become. Gather concrete tangible artifacts (photos, quotations, success stories) that you can use to imagine your own success.

1. Create your own mental film of what you want to look and feel like at your goal weight.
2. See yourself navigating self-control challenges and enjoying nutrient-dense food and exercise to achieve your goal.
3. Know and feel that your journey is empowering and powerful! Use the *Visualization Tips* table to help you achieve your own goals.

VISUALIZATION TIPS
Use all your senses
Be the star and the audience
Practice
Record via journal, audio or video
Be very specific
Visualize each step in process, not just the end result or product
Enjoy the journey
Include a pragmatic appraisal of your situation. Be positive but realistic.

8

Document Your Journey

Getting from point A to point Z can be daunting
unless you remember that you don't have to get from A to Z.
You just have to get from A to B.
Breaking big dreams into small steps is the way
to move forward.
~ SHERYL SANDBERG

We strongly believe that both speaking and writing about most issues in life help us to understand, evaluate, and if necessary, redirect our thoughts, beliefs, and behaviors. A daily entry in a weight-loss journal can do all of this as well as equip you to get a grip on issues about your weight. We agree with Julia Cameron, author of *The Writing Diet*, when she states, "Writing makes us conscious." In addition to writing, documenting your journey in any form such as photographs, recordings, and drawings will facilitate weight-loss.

Journaling focuses on establishing goals as well as planning manageable activities to achieve your goals. Every week I created a food and activity plan as well as strategies, including implementation intentions for handling any upcoming challenges. I reviewed my plans daily.

It's easier to evaluate your progress if you document what you eat, do, think, and feel each day. I got in the habit of monitoring my behavior by writing down *everything that I ate*. Since a major objective of journaling is to understand your behaviors, I kept notes on my hunger, thirst, and emotions in daily entries. I wrote detailed entries for the first sixty days of my weight-loss plan as I dug the trench for new behaviors. For me, it was important to record both quantifiable data such as weight, menus, and nutritional values, as well as qualitative information such as thoughts and feelings.

My journal entries were written in a conversant and stream-of-consciousness style as I tried to record specific facts as well as what I was thinking throughout the day. I was obsessive about only one thing...I had to write in my journal *every day*, knowing that writing would push me to a higher degree of awareness.

Writing forces you to answer questions about yourself that you might otherwise overlook or ignore. It enables you to be subjective when writing about your emotions and then objective when you are analyzing and reframing (looking at a situation from a different perspective) and redirecting (establishing new patterns of behaviors). You're basically a participant-observer of your mental processes. When you read your journals, you can check for faulty thinking, negative self-talk, and counter-productive cognitive distortions.

We'd always read that journaling is important, but now we have first-hand proof that written self-monitoring is one of the most effective strategies for changing behavior.

Research has shown that if people consistently take notes throughout the day, they will begin to notice their automatic responses and begin to eat differently. We already mentioned journaling as a simple yet powerful tool to shed light on our automatic behaviors. In fact, keeping a journal can double a person's weight loss. In one study, the most powerful predictor of weight loss was how many days per week a person wrote down what they ate. That's one powerful tactic.

In addition to journaling, I monitored and documented my progress in a variety of other ways. I took self-photos every two weeks and made audio and video recordings. For me, it was important to have documentation of my progress as well as an accurate view of what I looked like and how I was feeling. My journals, photos, and audio and videotape documentation had a huge impact on my success. I could no longer hide my weight or feelings in a cardboard box. As an educator, I've observed the importance of establishing, reinforcing, and supplementing an idea with visual aids to maximize an audience's understanding. Now I recognize the value of using visual aids for my own self-monitoring.

As I got closer to my goal weight, my journal entries became fewer and briefer as my new and healthier behavior became more automatic. Be patient because a change of habit can take anywhere from 66 to 250 repetitions of the new behavior. Just know that journaling is a great way to establish new behaviors.

Change of habit = 66 to 250 repetitions

WEIGH YOURSELF

When I was heavier, I seldom weighed myself because I didn't want to attach a negative label to my identity. I suppose that a lack of a benchmark made it easier to slide down the slippery slope of weight gain. In addition, when I wasn't on an official diet, I never kept track of my caloric or nutritional intake and I did my best to escape from negative and unsettling emotions. The reality was hidden from my awareness.

For me, it became motivating to weigh-in to monitor my progress. At first, I had to force myself to get on the scale once a week. In the past, if my weight went up, I'd be disappointed and jump off the wagon. This time around, armed with perseverance and a clear goal, I bit the bullet and decided that a daily weigh-in was nonnegotiable. I relabeled my weight as a number on a scale that provided an important benchmark of success. Detaching from the emotions surrounding the number on a scale provided a more objective and healthier view of my journey.

As a form of monitoring, weighing is a personal choice that can be motivating. A 2015 study showed that people who weighed themselves daily lost significantly more weight compared with those who weighed themselves less often. However, other studies showed that monitoring of the *process* of habit formation, rather than the outcome, was associated with success. The *process* – for example, eating three healthy meals each day – is the top priority. Both process and outcome can be tracked by journaling.

About half-way into my weight loss, I found a website where I could record my diet and weight as well as graph my progress. By objectifying, detaching, and compartmentalizing from the numbers on the scale, which could vary depending on my intake of salt or water as well as exercise, I weighed and recorded my weight every day. Now I weigh myself every week and if I exceed my target weight, I'll adjust my behavior.

Documenting my thoughts, behaviors, and habits through journaling, photographs, and audio/video recording was imperative for getting in touch with my eating, thoughts, and patterns. It's a tool that can help you to find your own truth.

IMPLEMENTATION

Document Your Journey is the sixth scientific principle of weight-loss success. Use journaling and recording to establish a benchmark, cognitively defuse and reframe maladaptive thoughts and behaviors, and document progress.

1. Write a prescriptive plan explaining how you will achieve your weight loss goals. Make sure that your goals and supporting activities are written in specific, measurable, attainable, realistic, and time-based terms.
2. Document your thoughts, feelings, behaviors, and progress through written text and media sources (audio, video, etc.). Record what you eat, your physical activities, and your emotional reactions to cues and triggers. A journal is the place to get in touch with your thoughts, feelings, and behaviors. The adage "A picture is worth a thousand words" has a great deal of merit so utilize images that are meaningful to you. The following *Journal Entry* will provide insight about journaling.

JOURNAL ENTRY	
Date:	
Weight:	
Breakfast:	Greek Yogurt with Chia Seeds Tortilla with Almond Butter Banana Black Tea
Lunch:	Romaine Salad with Oil & Rice Vinegar Dressing Seed Crackers with Minced Vegetables & Hummus Almonds Peppermint Tea
2 p.m.	After working at computer & feeling stressed, I felt like going out to buy a treat (sugar/chocolate). Decided to wait for 20 minutes, drink water, & eat vegetable soup. I took a brief walk after eating soup to get away from the computer and reinforce the notion that I'm happiest when I can balance work, exercise, and healthy eating. After eating something healthy & waiting, I didn't run out for hyperpalatable food. Way to go!
Dinner:	Soy Cheeseburger with Kosher Dill Pickle, Veggies, & Baked Fries Celery with Peanut Butter Lemonade (homemade, sweetened with Stevia)
Exercise:	3 mile brisk walk before breakfast Reached 10,000 steps for day 10 minutes of yoga stretching for flexibility
Comments:	Found a new path for walking. It's good to see and hear new stimuli on walk! Drank over 15 cups of water today as I was sweating on my brisk walk! I was thirsty. Posted new photos of hikers on difficult trails on my vision board. See it to be it!

9

Practice Compassion

A moment of self-compassion can change your entire day.
A string of such moments can change the course of your life.
~ CHRISTOPHER K. GERMER

We've all experienced times when we needed to think outside of the box to find a solution to a problem or challenge. The strategy that I used the last time I was stuck was to take a close look at my mental scripts. Sometimes our subconscious scripts keep us stuck because of faulty thinking or as a result of automatic habits of thought. One way to find your truth is through the examination of your self-talk.

Self-talk is also referred to as internal conversation, inner voice, internal dialogue, or inner dialogue. Self-talk is basically what we tell ourselves about ourselves and our world. In the field of psychology, many therapies use metacognition or *thinking about thinking* to overcome negative behaviors. When I analyzed my journals, I found that I had a habit of automatically labeling myself as a failure if I overate or didn't stick to someone else's prescribed diet plan. I was critical of *myself*, rather than the *act* of overeating, and thus my negative labeling was untrue, unnecessary, and nonproductive.

Like many people, I was critical in my conscious and unconscious thoughts about my eating. This is not unusual as research indicates that most people say hundreds of things to themselves each day and many may be negative self-talk statements. The key lies in being mindful of our inner dialogue so that we achieve accurate and supportive self-talk. Our self-talk can be extremely valuable OR detrimental to the success of healthy eating. If you're constantly telling yourself that you'll never lose weight, that you'll always be out of shape, that your genes are the culprit of your inability to lose weight, or that you'll start a new diet next Monday, you may talk yourself into a series of negative behaviors and never achieve what you want. When it comes to self-talk, realistic and positive thoughts lead to positive behaviors.

When examining your self-talk, look for cognitive distortions that may negatively affect your attitude and behavior. Cognitive distortions are ways that we convince ourselves of something that may, in fact, be untrue. Cognitive distortions are automatic statements that aren't productive or correct. If you see yourself and your behaviors in all-or-nothing terms, such as "I am overweight now so I'll never be thin," you are using irrational and incorrect thinking. The key is to analyze your thoughts to determine if there is truth in them. If you find that you're using a cognitive distortion, then refute and correct your thinking.

Many mental health practitioners including psychiatrist Aaron Beck and Dr. David Burns, psychologist and author of *Feeling Good: The New Mood Therapy*, have written about cognitive distortions that can keep us stuck. People may unconsciously use these distortions and limit their chance of weight loss success. For many dieters, the thought that "I ate one piece of pie, so I'll just eat the whole thing" is the familiar "what-the-hell" effect as well as the all-or-nothing cognitive distortion. It is a consequence of a rigid, zero-tolerance approach to weight loss. When I reviewed my journals, I found that I used *All-or-nothing thinking* (I ate one chocolate so I'll just overeat) as well as *'Should' statements* (I should start a diet on Monday) and *Labeling* (I'm gross if I don't lose weight.)

Cognitive reframing is a psychological technique that consists of identifying and then disputing irrational or maladaptive thoughts that are counterproductive to weight loss. Reframing is a way of viewing and experiencing events, ideas, concepts and emotions from a rational and positive perspective. Once you identify irrational beliefs such as cognitive distortions, you can use cognitive reframing to change your automatic thinking.

About 50 pounds ago, I used to think that it was almost impossible to lose weight. Once I reframed the thought to a more truthful and positive statement – "It's empowering and powerful to lose weight" – I was more inclined to exhibit behavior that reinforced my belief.

If you have a habit of using cognitive distortions, you may need to balance the scales. Throughout my weight loss, I became increasingly mindful of my thoughts as I recorded internal dialogue that needed to be altered, eliminated, or reinforced.

POSITIVE EMOTIONS ACCELERATE WEIGHT LOSS

Dr. Kristin Neff, author of *Self-Compassion: The Proven Power of Being Kind to Yourself*, states, "Many people believe that they need to be self-critical to motivate themselves, but in fact they just end up feeling anxious, incompetent and depressed. Far from encouraging self-indulgence, self-compassion helps us to see ourselves clearly and make needed changes because we care about ourselves and want to reach our full potential."

When we recognize our own imperfections and slipups without getting caught up in negative emotions, we increase the chances of self–regulation in the future. Dr. Neff explains that self-compassion has three components: being kind and understanding toward oneself in instances of pain or failure rather than being harshly self-critical; perceiving one's experiences as part of the larger human experience rather than seeing them as isolating; and holding painful thoughts and feelings in mindful awareness rather than over-identifying with them.

> *With self-kindness, we soothe and calm our troubled minds.*
> *We make a peace offering of warmth, gentleness and*
> *sympathy from ourselves to ourselves,*
> *so that true healing can occur.*
> ~ DR. KRISTIN NEFF

Whereas negative emotions of all kinds are linked to out-of-control eating and obesity positive emotions are linked to creative thinking skills, coping skills, and weight loss. Compassion can initiate an upward spiral of positive thoughts and emotions which can help you to fulfill your goals. To accelerate weight loss, resolve to treat yourself with loving kindness as you would a dear friend. Know that you're training your mind to see and think differently and that negative self-talk does not equate with failure. The goal is to become aware of our inner voice, correct statements if they are not true, change behaviors if necessary, and truly become our own good friend.

For me, an important part of compassion also involves cultivation of kindness for others. As discussed in an article in *Scientific American*, many studies have noted the positive effects of love and kindness thinking. "According to the Buddhist contemplative tradition from which this practice is derived, compassion, far from leading to distress and discouragement, reinforces an inner balance, strength of mind, and a courageous determination to help those who suffer." Compassion helped me to cultivate an inner strength that enabled me to succeed in my weight-loss efforts.

IMPLEMENTATION

Practice Compassion is the seventh scientific principle of weight-loss success. Weight loss entails an honest self-appraisal of our habits, thoughts, and behaviors as well as an expression of compassion for ourselves and others. Use the following *Cognitive Reframing* table to shift toward a healthier thought process.

COGNITIVE REFRAMING	
Cognitive reframing is a psychological technique that consists of identifying and then disputing irrational or maladaptive thoughts that are counterproductive to weight loss. Here are a few irrational thoughts that have been reframed.	
OLD	**NEW**
Hyperpalatable foods are rewards. The more, the better.	Healthy nutrient-dense foods are rewards for my body, mind, and soul.
I'll never lose weight unless I starve.	Losing weight can involve eating a lot of delicious foods.
It's no fun to lose weight.	It's fun, empowering, and powerful to lose weight.

1. Analyze your self-talk each day and reframe any nonproductive thoughts.
2. Create five ways that you can express compassion for others and yourself. What effect does compassion have on your thoughts, moods, and behaviors?

10

Reduce Stress

Calmness is the cradle of power.
~ J.G. HOLLAND

For years, people have suspected that stress and weight gain are linked — now research supports this connection. Approximately 50% of people who are concerned with stress cope by engaging in unhealthy behaviors including smoking, using alcohol or drugs, and overeating. Chronic life stress is associated with a greater appetite and desire for hyperpalatable foods. When I reflect on my heavier days, I recognize that overeating was a common way to deal with stress. So if you tend to cope with stress and other negative emotions by overeating or binge eating, you are not alone.

Everybody experiences stress and negative emotions to various degrees. The first key to decreasing stress is to recognize when and how it manifests in our lives. Then we need to work on reducing and preventing stress through proven and proactive strategies such as mindfulness, deep breathing, physical activity, and self-compassion.

Stress-management methods have been proven to boost weight loss. Proven stress-relievers include exercise and sports, yoga or tai chi, friendships, creative activities, contact with nature, music, meditation, and deep breathing. Women in one study who experienced the *greatest reduction in stress* tended to have the *most loss* of abdominal fat. This suggests that stress reduction should be a goal in itself, a part of every weight-loss plan, and a component of a new, healthier lifestyle. Let's examine the way in which deep breathing and physical activity can help you reduce stress and lose weight.

REDUCE STRESS THROUGH DEEP BREATHING

Deep breathing directly counters the effects of stress and it builds self-control if it is practiced regularly. Buddhist monks and meditation practitioners have known about the power of breathing for centuries. The effect is real and it is based in physiology. In the Western world, psychologists are beginning to incorporate the technique in advanced stress-reduction programs.

To understand how controlled breathing can be beneficial, first consider what happens when we encounter a stressful situation at work or at home. The body responds to stress by activating the fight-or-flight response. Our heart rate and breathing speed up and prepare us for action. A measurement known as heart rate variability or HRV is a good indicator of the flight-or-flight response. HRV refers to the variation in the intervals between heartbeats. Too little variation indicates stress, panic, anxiety, or worry.

The fight-or-flight response is physiologically linked to the "hot" system of the brain. In times of stress, the "hot" system takes over and the "cool" system, which resides in the prefrontal cortex, goes offline. As a result, stress has a detrimental effect when it comes to rational thinking, decision making, visualizing the future, and resisting temptations. If we can counteract this response, we can restore self-control.

The opposite of the fight-or-flight response has been called the *pause-and-plan* response by Dr. Suzanne Segerstrom. You take a deep breath and your body relaxes, giving you time for more thoughtful action. Instead of your heart speeding up, it slows down. By deliberately slowing the breath to around six breaths per minutes, compared with an average breathing rate of about 12 to 18 breaths a minute, we can shift the brain and body to a state of calm, thereby restoring self-control.

The fascinating part of the story is that the regulation of heart rate and breathing resides in the *same region of the brain* as self-control. This explains why slow breathing and meditation, which reduce stress, also strengthen self-control. Positive and negative emotions also are reflected in the pattern of the heart's rhythm. You can positively influence your own HRV by placing your attention in the center of your chest and creating a feeling of calmness, serenity, or contentment. The practice of self-compassion has a positive impact on HRV.

> *Feelings come and go like clouds in a windy sky.*
> *Conscious breathing is my anchor.*
> ~ THICH NHAT HANH, AUTHOR OF
> *STEPPING INTO FREEDOM:*
> *RULES OF MONASTIC PRACTICE FOR NOVICES*

In clinical settings, HRV is often measured with an electrocardiogram or ECG. However, anyone can monitor their own HRV with a hand-held device designed for that purpose, making biofeedback possible. In a study of individuals who frequently experienced food cravings, twelve sessions of HRV biofeedback reduced cravings. Importantly, HRV is an index that is directly associated with weight-loss success in dieters.

For anyone who wants to gain control over their environment or their emotions, slow breathing and HRV biofeedback are powerful techniques that can strengthen self-control *before* temptation strikes. There are videos on the Web that are designed to guide slow or "resonant" breathing, as well as more sophisticated biofeedback technologies that enable you to optimize your own personal HRV. This does not require hours of practice. Like most habits, it just requires repetition. The regular practice of this technique can help you buffer the stress in your life, boost self-control, feel happier, and lose weight.

REDUCE STRESS THROUGH PHYSICAL ACTIVITY

Physical activity is an excellent way to reduce stress, anxiety, and negative emotions. It even counteracts the cellular aging that is linked to chronic stress. In a review of long-term weight-loss success, physical activity was included in 88% of successful strategies. Research demonstrates that physical activity helps to control weight *and* to reduce the risk of heart disease, diabetes, and other medical conditions. Unfortunately, 79% of American adults don't meet U.S. guidelines for exercise. The guidelines recommend *at least* 2 ½ hours of moderate activity, such as brisk walking, every week.

Physical activity promotes feelings of well-being, boosts self-control, and diminishes reward-driven eating. Physical activity has a domino effect: by enhancing your mood, it increases your ability to tackle life's challenges – including dietary changes – with enthusiasm and optimism. In their book *Exercise for Mood and Anxiety,* Drs. Michael Otto and Jasper Smits write that doing any type of exercise on a regular basis makes people feel better about their bodies.

Always consult a physician before starting any exercise program. I began my regular physical activity by walking each morning. I timed myself and then set an objective of increasing my time and speed each week. I have a friend who started her exercise regimen by walking around her neighborhood. Now she walks about 3 miles each day.

In the beginning of my weight-loss journey, I utilized visualization by creating a mental picture of myself participating in a 5K run, climbing a difficult mountain, and experiencing the joy I had when I was bicycle riding and swimming as a youth. Last January, I replaced my virtual film with actual photographs of myself participating in a race, hiking up the very same mountain, and biking. My visualization was replaced with photos and feelings that were far more pleasurable than those I'd ever experienced when overeating. I've never regretted any time that I've spent participating in physical activity.

About one month into my activity regimen, I started keeping track of the number of steps I took each day. Setting an objective of 10,000 steps per day, I recorded my steps with a pedometer. There is a plethora of electronic devices that record your movement and provide immediate feedback on an iPhone, iPad, or computer. You can increase your steps by parking as far away from a store as possible, taking the stairs instead of an elevator, and getting up and moving after 45 minutes of sitting.

Make it easy to go walking by setting out your clothes and planning your walking path the night before. Whenever or whatever exercise you plan, schedule it in your calendar as a non-negotiable time when you will take care of yourself through movement. Just decide that you will schedule and follow through with physical activity. To form the good habit of regular exercise, avoid excuses and exercise every day.

Whether you're trying to develop a habit of journaling or physical activity, focus on the present moment one day at a time. Although you have vivid, long-term goals in mind, *success* lies in getting up Monday morning and practicing a new habit. And then doing the same thing on Tuesday, Wednesday, and so on. The more often you repeat the activity in the same context, the faster it will become automatic, and the more weight you can lose. Missing a day once in a while does not mean the end of the fledgling habit, so don't beat yourself up – just get back to it as soon as possible.

Scientific studies have shown that it takes months to change long-standing habits such as eating behaviors. With repetition, actions that are initially difficult to stick to become easier to maintain, and they ultimately become second nature. As you keep track of your behaviors through journaling you can note how automatic or natural the new behavior feels. Remember that our brains are designed to form new habits, and that it just requires patience and persistence to make the change.

Movement, deep breathing and other activities help to reduce stress and negative emotions while boosting your energy level and facilitating weight loss. The goal is simply to make physical activity and other healthy behaviors a habit.

We can use decision-making to choose the habits
we want to form,
use willpower to get the habit started,
then – and this is the best part –
we can allow the extraordinary power of habit to take over.
~ GRETCHEN RUBIN

IMPLEMENTATION

Reduce Stress is the eighth scientific principle of weight-loss success.

For many people, overeating is a common automatic coping mechanism for dealing with stress. Once you understand stress and its effect on your weight, you can break the cycle. Use the following *Healthy Habits Reduce Stress* table to examine your own habits.

HEALTHY HABITS REDUCE STRESS	
Deep breathing	
Meditation	
Exercise	
Walking	
Tai Chi	
Sports	
Yoga	→ **REDUCE STRESS** → **WEIGHT LOSS**
Music	
Humor	
Friendships	
Adequate sleep	
Creative activities	
Contact with nature	

1. Discuss at least five stressors in your life as well as how you cope with them.
2. Find a new coping mechanism each week. Try a new form of physical activity or hobby, write in your journal, or just wait it out. There're your stressors so identify the best way to deal with them. Focus on achieving a calm and healthy balance.

11

Delay Gratification

Thoughts lead on to purposes;
purposes go forth in action;
actions form habits;
habits decide character;
and character fixes our destiny.
~ TYRON EDWARDS

The world holds an abundance of foods that tempt us to indulge in immediate gratification. Our co-worker arrives with a box of doughnuts, we smell cinnamon rolls at the mall or airport, and/or the dessert table at a buffet calls our name. Life poses many self-control challenges.

Our attraction to high-sugar/high-fat foods stems from the physiological, psychological and cultural association of hyperpalatable foods with rewards. Temptations simultaneously create an immediate desire for indulgence, while conflicting with our long-term weight-loss goals. Many people end up in a mental tug-of-war between what they want now, such as the immediate gratification of a chocolate chip cookie, and what they want in the future, such as the delayed gratification of a slimmer body.

What determines whether we will give in to temptation or resist? The answer is determined by a competition between the impulsive or "hot" system in the brain, which was discussed in Chapter 4, and the rational or "cool" system. In the face of strong temptations, the "hot" system reacts instantaneously, before we are aware of the impulse, and prompts us to give in. When this occurs we need to intervene quickly by removing ourselves from the temptation or remaining inactive until the "hot" signal subsides.

More than 40 years ago, Dr. Walter Mischel began to study how children handled a similar dilemma. Mischel discusses the studies in his book, *The Marshmallow Test*. Here's how the test was done: one by one, children were brought into a room and were told they could have one marshmallow immediately, while a researcher left the room. However, if they could wait until the researcher returned, they could have two marshmallows.

As you can imagine, some children chose the immediate reward of a single marshmallow over the longer-term reward of two marshmallows. Other children came up with creative ways to resist the immediate reward, for example by looking away from the marshmallow or singing a song.

Thirty years later, researchers caught up with the children who took the original Marshmallow Test and evaluated their body mass index or BMI as adults. They found that the preschoolers who were able to delay gratification had *lower body weights* as adults as compared with those who succumbed right away. In fact, each additional minute that a preschooler delayed gratification predicted a 0.2-point reduction in BMI in adulthood. It was a simple test with profound implications for weight loss and other self-control challenges. In one of our favorite stories from *The Marshmallow Test*, Mischel asks a child, "What's self-control?" The child answers: "It's *thinking* before *doing*."

Self-Control = Thinking Before Doing

HOW CAN YOU GET MORE SELF-CONTROL?
Throughout this book, we've included tactics to boost self-control including proactive avoidance of high-sugar/high-fat foods, the use of implementation intentions, mindfulness, journaling, reducing stress, delaying in the face of cravings, embracing nutrient-dense foods, and reframing the value of short-term rewards versus long-term rewards. As Dr. Mischel

says: "The core strategy for self-control is to cool the NOW and heat the LATER: push the temptation in front of you far away in space and time, and bring the distant consequences closer in your mind."

So how do we boost our self-control? Review and utilize the tactics we've discussed so far. Consider these examples of ways to stay in the moment, delay immediate gratification (cool the NOW) and promote long-term gratification (heat the LATER):

- Visualize your future. Focus on the long-term consequences of hyperpalatable foods such as candy, cake, pizza, or French fries to reduce cravings for those foods.
- "Bring to life" your dreams and visions through visualization. When we envision ourselves actually wearing the clothes we want to wear, looking healthy and attractive in a slimmer body, it helps us focus on the long-term reward.
- Get moving. Physical activity improves mood and self-efficacy.
- Reduce stress. Stress reduction techniques boost self-control.
- Practice mindfulness and resonant breathing to activate the pause-and-plan response.
- Practice self-compassion as it counteracts black-and-white thinking.
- Proactively avoid high-sugar/high-fat foods to prevent reward-driven eating.
- Use implementation intentions to deal with triggers and cues in order to persist with your goals.
- Tune out food advertisements and displays as this puts you back in the driver's seat.
- Prepare and plan meals with tasty, nutrient-dense foods that provide the joy of trying new tastes, the afterglow of better digestion, and the sense of accomplishment that comes from creating a meal that is not only good tasting but good for you.

- Take one step at a time. Every instance of successful planning and implementation contributes to short-term satisfaction through avoiding and dealing with motivational conflict – the kind of conflict that comes with thinking one thing (*I want to lose weight*) and doing another (*I can't resist those doughnuts.*)

IMPLEMENTATION

Delay Gratification is the ninth scientific principle of weight-loss success. Be aware that you're changing your behavior by delaying gratification. There's power in turning an immediate, automatic reaction into a mindful response by *thinking before doing*. Reflect on the following Delay Gratification table.

DELAY GRATIFICATION
When a stimulus (cue or trigger) surfaces, what are you going to do?
CHANGE:
Stimulus → **Reaction** (eating hyperpalatable food)
TO:
Stimulus → Delayed Reaction → **Response**
BY IMPLEMENTING:
Mindfulness
Waiting
Exercise

1. Through journaling, make note of the self-control challenges you commonly identify each week at work, home, the market, restaurants, and other environments. Note when and where the self-control challenges occur.
2. Review the *Implementation Intentions* table in Chapter 5 to tailor your environment to fit your goals.
3. Use the *Should I Eat This?* Table in Appendix B to create your own set of governing questions to ask yourself before you overeat.

4. Write about your views of high-sugar/high-fat foods versus healthy foods and consider the long-term consequences of different types of foods. Are you ready and willing to focus on long-term gratification rather than immediate gratification?

12

Focus on Nutrient-Dense Foods

Changing the whole world is overwhelming,
but changing our personal food radius is very doable.
~ DR. BRIAN WANSINK, AUTHOR OF *SLIM BY DESIGN*

M any weight loss books begin by discussing food menus, and yet we've placed our discussion of food in the next-to-last chapter. Why? Because it is important to understand *why we eat* before we can implement a successful weight loss plan.

We must acknowledge the impact of our environment, thoughts, feelings, behaviors, and habits on our eating patterns in order to make a change. Stress relief and dealing with emotional eating is an integral part of the process. It is easy to abuse hyperpalatable foods at any time and it is easy for our obesogenic environment to abuse us. Our plan focuses on becoming more aware, mindful, and proactive of external and internal eating triggers using all of the strategies we've described throughout this book.

An underlying principle in my transformation, as well as the basis of healthy eating, is that food, as Hippocrates stated over 2,000 years ago, is medicine. I read Hippocrates' words daily as a reminder that food is instrumental to wellbeing. It is empowering to know that you have the ability to alter your physical and emotional being through food. By believing and adopting Hippocrates' position that food is medicine, you can move in the right direction for a healthy existence.

Food = Medicine

A "DIET" DOES NOT REQUIRE EXTREME MEASURES

Fasting, severe calorie restriction, or the elimination of entire food groups are often the norm when it comes to dieting. Many weight loss plans focus on eating in an extreme way for a short period of time or they recommend a complex set of prescribed rules. We believe that the very concept of a diet as something involving extreme and externally imposed measures are two of the reasons weight-loss efforts fail.

Often people say, "I'm going on a diet." Immediately we think of some extremely restrictive eating plan. Yo-yo dieting involves going on an extreme diet, losing weight, going off the extreme diet and back to old habits, and gaining weight. And so forth and so on, *ad infinitum*.

It's true that one definition of a diet is "a special course of food to which one restricts oneself, either to lose weight or for medical reasons." However, another definition of a diet is "the kinds of food that a person habitually eats." Our point is that it's not necessary to consume *a special course of food* to lose weight. Instead, simply focus on the kinds of foods that you can eat to stay slim and healthy, and begin to eat that way *once and for all*. If you do this, your body will gradually approach your goal weight.

Here is how the calories worked for me.

Since I wanted to weigh 140 pounds, I needed to eat approximately 1600 calories per day to achieve and maintain that weight. When I first started eating fewer calories, my activity level was low and I was eating approximately 2200 calories per day so a new lifestyle meant reducing my daily caloric intake by approximately 600 calories per day.

By consuming 1600 calories of nutrient-dense foods per day, my weight gradually dropped until I weighed 140 pounds. When I ramped up my activity to a moderate level by walking every day I either lost weight faster or was able to consume more calories to continue losing weight.

Obviously, your target weight is whatever you and your doctor decide is right for you. Whatever your goal, you can find the daily calorie requirements for long-term maintenance in Appendix D. If you reduce your intake by 600 calories per day you will lose approximately one to two pounds per week, and if you increase your activity level you will lose weight faster.

Regarding activity, the American Heart Association recommends that we aim for at least 30 minutes of moderate physical activity on most days of the week or – best of all – at least 30 minutes each day. People who successfully maintain weight loss over the long term are those who incorporate exercise in their routine.

Now, let's examine the foods we need for long-term health.

TOO MANY CALORIES, NOT ENOUGH NUTRIENTS

Today, as in the past, a gap exists between what we are consuming and what we need for good health. High-sugar/high-fat products have squeezed nutrient-dense foods out of our diets. The U.S. diet contains too many calories and not enough vegetables, fruits, high-fiber whole grains, seafood, and low-fat milk products. As a result, many of us are not consuming enough folate, magnesium, potassium, dietary fiber, and vitamins A, C, and K. This is the consensus of the US Department of Agriculture and Health and Human Services. Every five years the agencies issue a report titled *Dietary Guidelines for Americans.*

The 2010 and 2015 *Dietary Guidelines* state that Americans consume too many calories from solid fats, added sugars, and refined grains, along with too much sodium. Alarming as it is, "64% of women and 72% of men are overweight or obese," "many Americans are unaware of how many calories they need each day or the calorie content of foods and beverages," and "very few Americans consume diets that meet dietary guidelines." Moreover, poor diet and inactivity are associated with major causes of morbidity and mortality such as cardiovascular diseases, type 2 diabetes, osteoporosis, and some types of cancer. That's the bad news. What's the good news? As individuals, we have the power to shift our course. We just have to take the plunge.

You can't eat junk food and expect to live an unjunked life.
You are what you eat, what you believe, what you do.
~ O MAGAZINE

Prior to my weight loss, I consumed too many calories from unhealthy foods, I was overweight, and I was unaware of the recommended nutritional guidelines for my age and gender. Our research indicates that I'm not alone in my ignorance of nutrition. In surveys of average Americans, a majority of respondents were unable to identify their daily nutritional requirements. Furthermore, the more knowledgeable I became about my nutritional requirements, the more likely I was to choose healthy foods when I cooked. Knowledge is power when it comes to selecting a healthy diet.

The *Dietary Guidelines* present two overarching concepts: 1) We need to maintain calorie balance to sustain a healthy weight and 2) Our diets should consist of nutrient-dense foods that have lots of nutrients but relatively few calories. The American Heart Association, the Harvard School of Public Health, the Mayo Clinic, and the Academy of Nutrition and Dietetics all recommend a diet based on nutrient-dense foods.

Nutrient-dense foods can be found in the five major food groups: 1) vegetables, 2) fruits, 3) whole grains, 4) healthy protein sources such as chicken, fish, beans, and legumes, and 5) low-fat dairy products. Needless to say, these foods are not found in the chips, soda and candy aisles or in most fast food restaurants.

Cutting out empty calories and high-sugar/high-fat foods, while focusing on nutrient-dense foods, is the basis of most healthy eating plans and of *The 20 Billion Dollar Diet*. Here's why nutrient-dense foods provide a solid basis for weight loss:

(1) Nutrient-dense foods provide the nutrition your body needs for optimal health, digestion, and energy.
(2) If you substitute nutrient-dense foods for nutrient-poor foods, you will be cutting calories.
(3) Fruits, vegetables, and whole grains are high in fiber. They boost satiety so you will not go hungry while you are losing weight.
(4) Nutrient-dense foods do not trigger out-of-control eating. You can eat them without stressing about overeating.

(5) A focus on preparing three nutrient-dense meals a day is readily aligned with the way in which habits are formed – one day at a time.

(6) Spending time on the preparation of nutrient-dense and satisfying meals facilitates mindful eating instead of mindless overeating.

MANY EATING PATTERNS WORK

The 20 Billion Dollar Diet does not advocate one type of eating pattern such as Mediterranean, vegetarian, or vegan as we concur with the *Dietary Guidelines for Americans* statement that "Many traditional eating patterns can provide health benefits, and their variety demonstrates that people can eat healthfully in a number of ways." The Academy of Nutrition and Dietetics affirms that "The total diet or overall pattern of food eaten is the most important focus of healthy eating."

What we do advocate is becoming informed about nutrient-dense guidelines so that you can make your own choices and decisions to satisfy your nutritional requirements.

Like most long-term dieters without an eating plan, I'll eat just about anything. Since I know this about myself, I plan out a week's worth of daily menus focused on nutrient-dense foods. During my weight loss journey I religiously wrote down my planned menus as well as what I actually ate. For the first 60 days I evaluated the nutrient content of everything so that I would meet my daily nutritional requirements. It was a great way to establish a quantifiable account of my behaviors.

Here are essential components of *The 20 Billion Dollar Diet* food plan.

REAL FOODS

The first step in eating well is to focus on real food. That means that you don't have to understand chemistry to know what you are eating. Foods need to be in their most natural state. For example, it's better to eat apples rather than drink apple juice. Cleanse your palate and acclimate your taste buds to non-industrial, non-processed foods that don't contain artificial ingredients. I found that I like celery with hummus, apples, nuts, berries, bananas, and spinach in their natural states.

I ate very simply, eating as close to the natural state of the food as possible. I gave up all sodas, diet sodas, chips, chocolate, candy, and other artificial and processed foods. When I read that Americans are eating 500 calories more now than in the 1970s due to high-calorie, high-sugar/high-fat snacks, and that sugar triggers overeating, I stopped my weekly visits to convenience stores, fast-food restaurants, and pastry shops. At the super-market, I avoided the candy, cookie and chip aisles.

While many of us grew up disliking vegetables, all of my favorite recipes now include vegetables. If you think you won't like vegetables or you anticipate a bitter taste, try delicious sliced oven-roasted vegetables such as carrots, cauliflower, zucchini, red bell peppers, beets, tomatoes, mushrooms, sweet potatoes, and squash brushed with a bit of olive oil. Oven-roasting transforms vegetables by caramelizing the natural sugar within them and creating a toasty flavor. When freshly roasted with a little salt and pepper or herbs, vegetarian fare is at the top of our "Nutrient-Dense and Tasty" list.

> *Don't eat anything your great-grandmother wouldn't*
> *recognize as food.*
> ~ MICHAEL POLLAN

WHAT ABOUT SUGAR?

I used to eat hyperpalatable comfort foods that had large amounts of sugar and fat. When eating these foods became a habitual eating pattern with subsequent weight and health issues, I eliminated high-sugar/high-fat foods, resetting my palate to enjoy fruits and vegetables.

Beverages that contain added sugar are major contributors to obesity. Juice often contains as much sugar and as many calories as sugary soda, and unlike fruit, juice is not a good source of fiber. Although many dieters go for calorie-free sodas, there is growing concern that certain artificial sweeteners may have negative effects on long-term health.

The U.S. Department of Agriculture (USDA) and the World Health Organization recommend limiting added sugar to 25 grams per day. The

American Heart Association points out that it is fine to use a small amount of sugar, if needed, to improve the taste of healthy foods such as fruit, yogurt, or whole grain cereal.

The recommendation for limiting sugar does not apply to the fructose that is naturally present in whole fruits, or to the lactose that is naturally present in low-fat dairy products. These naturally occurring substances are accompanied by fiber (in fruit) or protein (in yogurt), which slow digestion and do not trigger overeating. We've never known anyone to binge on fresh fruit or Greek yogurt. A bowl of fresh fruit topped with kefir makes an excellent alternative to traditional sugar-laden desserts.

I also found that I enjoy homemade lemonade sweetened with Stevia. Stevia is a virtually calorie-free natural sweetener extracted from the leaves of the plant species *Stevia rebaudiana*; it has been used for centuries as a sweetener in South America. Studies have shown that Stevia provides a level of satiety similar to that of sucrose (sugar), without the calories.

PLANT-BASED FOOD

A few years ago, I ran into a friend who I hadn't seen in a very long time. He looked younger and fitter than I remembered him. My friend told me that he had lost a lot of weight a couple of years before, but his cholesterol count remained high. He ended up lowering his cholesterol by adopting a plant-based diet. Before my weight loss, I had high cholesterol and a prescription for a cholesterol-lowering drug. After adopting a plant-based diet, my cholesterol is in the normal range.

According to Dr. Dean Ornish, the author of *Eat More, Weigh Less* and an advocate of a plant-based diet, "Our research proved that the progression of even severe heart disease often can be reversed by making comprehensive lifestyle changes. When you change your lifestyle, you change [the influence of] your genes." An annual physical exam and bloodwork provide benchmarks for determining any special dietary requirements or restrictions.

During my weight loss, I read several books and articles by Michael Pollan, a contributor to *The New York Times* and author of *Cooked* and *Food*

Rules. Cooked provides insight into humans' relationships with food, noting that while Americans are spending half as much time in the kitchen as we did in 1970, obesity rates are higher than ever before. When I was larger, I spent less time in the kitchen than I do now. As a vegetarian, I currently spend a lot of time chopping. I've thought about purchasing a food processor but for now, chopping is a mindful and meditative process for me. It makes me think about what I'm eating.

If you choose to eat meat, emphasize chicken and fish rather than red meat, and chow down on the veggies first. For weight loss and flavor you can add a low-calorie/low-fat dressing to vegetables and salads.

The USDA recommends eating fish twice a week to obtain heart-healthy omega-3 fatty acids. Salmon is a good source of omega-3 fatty acids, Vitamin D and Vitamin E. A different form of omega-3 fatty acids occurs in plants, and more plant omega-3s are needed to get the same heart health benefits as from fish. Good sources of plant omega-3s are flax seeds or chia seeds as well as raw walnuts.

YOGURT AND KEFIR

While I was growing up, I never liked or ate yogurt. In my heavier days, it was one of those foods that I'd eat if it was frozen and smothered in bits of chocolate or hot fudge: in short, if it tasted like ice cream. I started eating yogurt because of Marina, who advises that yogurt and/or kefir should be part of every diet, whether for weight loss or just for good health. My experience has supported Marina's belief and every morning I eat at least one container of Greek yogurt with other breakfast foods. Low fat Greek yogurt is a good source of protein, providing approximately 25% of the Recommended Dietary Allowance, or RDA, per serving. One serving of Greek yogurt also provides approximately 15% of the RDA for calcium.

In addition to protein and calcium and good flavor, yogurt is a cultured milk product that contains beneficial live bacteria, also known as probiotics, which keep your digestion humming along. Recent studies suggest that the balance of bacteria in our gut may help protect against obesity. Kefir, which is drinkable, has higher quantities of probiotic bacteria than yogurt. Kefir is delicious in smoothies.

Lactobacillus and *Bifidobacterium* are the main species of probiotic bacteria. *Lactobacillus* species are associated with immunity, while *Bifidobacterium* species have anti-inflammatory effects. In one study, people who live to be 100 years old were found to have *Bifidobacterium* populations comparable to those of younger individuals. All yogurts contain *Lactobacillus acidophilus*, but you have to look on the label for yogurt that contains *Bifidus*, the abbreviation for *Bifidobacterium*. Kefir is the best source of probiotic bacteria, containing up to 100 times as many live bacteria as most yogurts. Some friends and colleagues have told us that, since they began consuming kefir, their irritable bowel symptoms have disappeared.

Plain yogurt has about 12 grams of natural sugar per serving, in the form of lactose that is fermented. This amount of naturally-occurring sugar is not of concern. Even if you are lactose-intolerant, you may be able to consume yogurt. However, some brands and flavors of yogurt have more sugar than a candy bar as a result of added sugar. Check the labels before buying, and see if you can find a brand and flavor you like with less than 20 grams of total sugar per serving.

FIBER

Dietary fiber reduces the risk of developing heart disease, diabetes, diverticular disease, and constipation, and supports the growth of beneficial gut bacteria. While adults need approximately 30 grams of fiber per day (25 grams for women and 38 grams for men), most Americans eat less than half that amount.

The current Dietary Guidelines suggest that half of each meal plate contain vegetables and fruits. Higher concentrations of fiber are associated with greater weight loss. Four months into my weight loss, my gastroenterologist told me that healthy colons need lots of fiber, the kind you get in vegetables and fruits. In fact, he suggested that three-fourths of each meal plate should contain vegetables and fruits. Dr. Susan Roberts, a scientist at the USDA, believes that fiber is a cornerstone of weight control. According to a USDA article, "For losing weight, I recommend at least 40 grams of fiber per day," says Dr. Roberts.

There are two types of fiber: insoluble and soluble. Insoluble fiber, which does not dissolve in water, can help food move through your digestive system, promoting regularity and helping prevent constipation. Foods with insoluble fibers include whole wheat bread, whole grain couscous, brown rice, tomatoes, carrots, cucumbers and legumes such as chickpeas in hummus.

Soluble fiber, which dissolves in water, can help lower glucose levels as well as help lower blood cholesterol. Foods with soluble fiber include oatmeal, nuts, beans, lentils, apples and blueberries. One cup of lentils has about 15 grams of fiber, an apple has four grams of fiber, and one artichoke has about 10 grams of fiber. The fiber foods swell in your stomach as they absorb liquid so you also feel fuller after you eat them. At each meal, I try to eat fiber foods first.

The Academy of Nutrition and Dietetics recommends ramping up on fiber slowly, since increasing dietary fiber quickly can lead to bloating or gas in some people. The bacteria in your colon usually adjust within a few weeks. Fermented foods such as yogurt and kefir assist in the process.

PROTEIN

Two months into my diet, friends said that I looked healthy and younger. And yet, one day I woke up tired after a full eight hours of sleep. When I checked nutrient requirements, I realized that I was not eating enough protein. In fact, until I started this journey, I was unaware of how much protein I actually needed. Now I know that adult women need approximately 46 grams of protein every day; men need approximately 56 grams; and women who are pregnant or lactating need 71 grams of protein daily. Healthy sources of protein should be included in every diet. For satiety and nutrition, consume some protein at every meal.

Meat, poultry, fish, seafood, eggs, nuts, seeds, soy products and beans and peas make up the protein food group. Animal sources of protein contain all the essential amino acids. Beans and peas are excellent sources of vegetarian protein, and they're also included in the vegetable group for their fiber content and nutrient profile. Other protein sources, such as vegetables, grains, nuts and seeds, lack one or more essential amino acids. As a vegetarian, I need to eat a variety of protein-containing foods each day.

The Harvard School of Public Health encourages us to limit red meat and avoid processed meat. These products are high in saturated fat and can increase the risk of heart disease and weight gain when overconsumed. If you are a burger lover, you might want to try turkey burgers, salmon burgers, or soy burgers. For meat-containing diets, focus on poultry and fish and minimize red meats.

WHAT ABOUT WHEAT?
Whole grains are important sources of fiber and nutrients such as zinc, magnesium, and B vitamins. Fiber has been identified as a nutrient of public health priority. Only one out of ten Americans succeeds in meeting fiber recommendations of 25 to 38 grams per day. There's no reason to avoid wheat unless you have celiac disease, which is present in 1% of the population, or another type of gluten intolerance or allergy.

The current USDA food guide, which can be found at the ChooseMyPlate website, provides a visual depiction of grains as approximately one-fourth of the plate at every meal. Whole-grain requirements can be met with foods such as oatmeal, brown rice, barley, popcorn, and whole-grain breads and cereals. Wheat bread does not necessarily contain whole grains; many of the breads contain milled flour instead. Look for the word "whole" at the beginning of the ingredients list. If the product provides *at least* five grams of fiber per serving, it is a great source of fiber.

In general, 1 slice of bread, 1 cup of ready-to-eat cereal, or ½ cup of cooked brown rice or cooked cereal can be considered as 1 ounce equivalent from the Grains Group, and the recommendations call for three- to six-ounce equivalents. Whole grain cereal for breakfast, a whole-grain sandwich for lunch, and brown rice with dinner are ways to meet the grain requirement. Try a vegetarian whole-grain sandwich with olive oil and herbs as a spread, along with cucumbers, tomatoes and avocado – or try sundried tomato spread.

WHAT ABOUT DAIRY PRODUCTS?

The consumption of dairy products, and of calcium overall, is associated with a decreased risk of obesity. The Dietary Guidelines recommends that women and men over 19 years of age consume three cups of reduced-fat dairy products per day and that most dairy group choices should be fat-free or low-fat.

In addition to calcium, fortified low-fat dairy, soy and almond milks provide Vitamin D for strong bones. We agree with major medical and nutrition organizations and government agencies, which recommend low-fat milk and cheese because of their decreased saturated fat and calorie content.

WATER

To boost weight loss, don't drink your calories; just drink water. The Healthy Eating Plate, developed by Harvard University, encourages us to drink water, since it's naturally calorie free. Dehydration can wear a false mask of hunger and because I live in a hot climate, my water intake is *at least* 12 cups per day. Water is our beverage of choice, with added lemon or cucumber if you like, or herbal tea.

NUTRITIONAL REQUIREMENTS

Since I decided to eat approximately 1600 calories per day to achieve my goal weight, I based my plan on three meals per day, with each meal contributing approximately 500 calories. I'm sharing my own eating plan and one of my breakfast menus for illustration purposes, and as a source of ideas to launch you on your own journey. *This is not a menu you have to follow.* We urge you to experiment and create your own menus using my ideas as a springboard. For me, each day's menu contains the following types of foods:

- At least 3 cups or servings of raw or cooked vegetables. To obtain a broad range of micronutrients, consume a variety of different colors of vegetables. Some tasty options include lettuce, celery, beets, carrots, broccoli, cauliflower, peppers, peas, potatoes (including sweet potatoes), onions, cabbage, spinach, and tomatoes.
- 2 pieces of your favorite fruit, for example: berries, banana, apple, orange, lemon, grapefruit, grapes, cherries, plum, peach, pear, and pomegranate.
- Approximately 46 grams of protein, for example: 6 ounces of turkey or chicken or fish (46 grams); 1 cup Greek yogurt (12 grams); 1 cup milk (9 grams); 1 egg (3 grams). Protein also can be obtained from beans or peas (1 cup of bean soup = 2 ounce-equivalents of protein.)
- Since I chose a vegetarian diet, I consumed approximately 1 cup (cooked) or 200 calories of beans per day, choosing from black, pinto or kidney beans or chickpeas.
- To save calories, I consume a maximum of 2 pieces of whole-grain bread or other whole-grain product per day
- Approximately 50 grams of healthy fat in products such as olive oil (1 TBS equals 14 grams), avocado (1 cup equals 21 grams); sunflower seeds (1/4 cup equals 17 grams); walnuts (1/4 cup equals 13 grams).
- A spoonful of chia seeds or golden flaxseed meal as a vegetarian source of omega-3 fatty acids.

Nutritional requirements vary with age and gender, and increase with pregnancy and lactation. The ChooseMyPlate website (USDA) provides detailed guidelines.

Analyzing the macronutrients in your meals can be an interesting task. I ended up evaluating everything I ate on the basis of criteria that were important to me. As you can see in the Sample Menu below, foods are broken down according to their calories and macronutrients (carbohydrates, protein, sugar, fat) and fiber.

								SAMPLE MENU : THE CONTINENTAL BREAKFAST
FOOD	Amount	Calories	Carbs (g)	Protein (g)	Sugar (g)	Fat (g)	Fiber (g)	Comments
Greek yogurt	5.3 oz	120	19	12	15	0	1	Great for digestion and immunity. Pick a brand that lists *Bifidus* on the label.
with chia seeds	1 TBS	69	6	2	0	4	5	Chia seeds fill me up. Also try golden flaxseed meal.
Whole grain toast	1 slice	110	21	0	3	1.5	3	Provides fiber and vitamins. Choose whole-grain bread.
with no- trans-fat margarine	1 TBS	70	0	0	0	8	0	Margarine has less saturated fat than butter. Only use margarine with no trans fat.
Coffee	2 cups	0	0	0	0	0	0	Substitute decaf if you prefer.
with fat-free half & half	4 TBS	40	6	2	6	0	0	I love cream so this is a modified splurge.
Blueberries	1 cup	85	21	1	15	0	3.6	Anti-oxidant food; fruit serving.
	TOTAL	494	73	17	39	13.5	12.6	

Today there are several websites and mobile apps that will save you the problem of manually adding up the nutritional value of what you eat. The point of *The 20 Billion Dollar Diet* is for *you* to take charge, select foods, and plan out your meals.

IS VARIETY THE SPICE OF LIFE?
In order to cleanse my palate at the beginning of my weight-loss journey, I ate simply, consuming foods in their natural states. Raw vegetables and fruits, with small portions of protein, made up the majority of my meals. As time went on, I added more variety. I make dressing with all types of vinegars, such as balsamic, rice, and malt vinegar to reduce calories and boost

the zest. While earlier in my life I seasoned with only salt and pepper, I now have a plethora of spices and herbs to use for seasoning. I also rely on a variety of delicious teas and homemade lemonade, sweetened with Stevia, to stimulate my taste buds.

In addition to planning and preparing food, I focus on food presentation. Before my weight loss, I only used my special china dishes and linen napkins on holidays and other special occasions. Now I prepare an attractive display with china dishes, flowers, and pretty linens at every meal. My objective is to prepare an attractive visual display that will add to the joyful experience of eating healthy food. Suffice to say, variety is the spice of a good diet.

As you begin your own healthy eating plan, keep it simple. The most important element is to build on the habit of eating three meals per day of nutrient-dense foods. This means finding foods you really enjoy eating for breakfast, lunch and dinner. In the early stages of habit formation, it is important to consume regular meals in the same place and at the same time of day. Variety can come later, after the healthy eating habit is firmly established.

QUESTIONS BEFORE YOU EAT

Today, I know a food's nutritional value before I put it in my mouth. I keep an ongoing mental record throughout the day of what I've eaten as well as whether it satisfies the following six steps for eating healthy foods. If I can answer "yes" to the following questions, I feel good about putting the food in my mouth.

- Is this food real or does it contain unpronounceable chemicals and additives?
- Is this food plant-based? If not, have I eaten enough plant-based foods to meet my daily needs?
- Does this food contribute fiber to my 25 gram recommended intake?

- Does this food add protein so that I can achieve 46 grams to meet my recommended dietary allowance?
- Am I adding unnecessary sugar?
- How many calories are in this food? Does it make a healthy contribution to my daily 1600 calorie intake?

Eating to live well is simple and much more satisfying than losing yourself in palatable foods. When you follow Hippocrates' advice to eat healthy food, you will feel and look better, lose weight, and empower yourself in all aspects of your life. Enjoy the great taste of healthy foods!

Marina MacDonald, M.S., Ph.D. and Judith A. McManus, M.A.

IMPLEMENTATION

Focus on Nutrient-Dense Foods is the tenth scientific principle of weight-loss success.

Scientific studies and experience support the importance of a diet consisting of nutrient-dense foods. One of the kindest things that you can do for yourself is to fuel your body with healthy food. Use *The 20 Billion Dollar Diet® Grocery List* in Appendix A, *Should I Eat This?* in Appendix B, *What Does 100 Calories Look Like?* in Appendix C, and the *Daily Calorie Requirements for Weight Maintenance* in Appendix D as tools to create your own menus.

1. List the daily nutritional requirements and calories you need each day.
2. Create a ten-day menu (three meals per day) of nutrient-dense food. Schedule each meal at approximately the same time every day.

13

Seek Happiness

Happiness is not the absence of problems,
it's the ability to deal with them.
~ STEVE MARABOLI

Whether you've arrived at this chapter after reading the whole book, or jumped to this chapter because you are interested in happiness, we're glad you're here. We hope that *The 20 Billion Dollar Diet* will empower you not only to lose weight, but also to experience more happiness in your life.

As you might guess, researchers have found that weight loss can make people happier. In the largest study of individuals successful at long-term maintenance of their goal weight, nearly all members indicated that weight loss led to improvements in their level of energy, general mood, self-confidence, and physical health.

But happiness is not just something we should expect in the future, *after* we have accomplished our weight loss or other life goals. Happiness can be a direct, daily byproduct of the processes we've discussed in this book. For example, physical activity, self-compassion, deep breathing, mindfulness and cognitive reappraisal of challenges can help you switch from anxiety and stress to equanimity and happiness.

Self-regulation is concerned with setting goals, developing and enacting strategies to achieve those goals, appraising progress, and revising goals and strategies accordingly. Numerous studies indicate that self-regulation has a strong positive correlation with psychological health and happiness.

A recent study tracked the symptoms of depression in people who were trying to quit smoking and found that they were never happier than when they were being successful, for however long that was.

Actively navigating the challenges of life contributes to a personal sense of competence, autonomy and well-being. Each step we take toward our goals leads us a step closer to happiness. Just following through on a goal one day at a time, such as getting physical activity every day, provides a sense of accomplishment: *I can do this.* This may explain why focusing on the *process* of weight loss is as important as the *goal.*

When you embrace the process of change, you become an active agent and decision-maker in your own life, rather than a helpless subject of external forces. That's an empowering way to live.

IMPLEMENTATION

Rather than being something that we should expect in the future *after* we have accomplished our weight loss goals, happiness should be a direct, daily byproduct of the processes we've discussed in this book. We hope that the following *Seek Happiness* table will help you to create your own happiness.

SEEK HAPPINESS	
Scientific Statement	**My Experience**
Physical activity relieves anxiety and improves mood	*I went for a 20 minute walk with Marina this am and felt better.*
Mindfulness, meditation and resonant breathing promote well-being	*It's important to practice these behaviors at approximately the same time every day.*
Self-compassion counteracts black-and-white thinking	*I feel better when I am nice to myself; I like myself better when I'm nice to others.*
Implementation intentions boost self-efficacy. This contributes to psychological well-being and helps you to persist with your goals.	*Implementation intentions help me to plan my success.*

14

The 20 Billion Dollar Diet

Knowing is not enough; we must apply.
Willing is not enough; we must do.
~ JOHANN WOLFGANG VON GOETHE

Now that you're familiar with my journey and the supporting scientific research, it's time to implement *The 20 Billion Dollar Diet* by completing the exercises at the end of each chapter if you have not already done so.

Psychologist Carl Jung once said, "You are what you do, not what you say you'll do." I spent many years, a lot of money, and needless energy thinking, reading, researching, and talking about wanting to be thin without actualizing my vision. Once I decided that I could and would follow a healthy plan, my life changed. *Success begins with action.* I took action and so can you!

Every step, every activity, every movement brings you closer to your goal weight. Take the plunge by implementing your own plan! Here is a summary of the ten scientific principles of weight-loss success which are discussed throughout this book.

TEN SCIENTIFIC PRINCIPLES of
WEIGHT-LOSS SUCCESS

BELIVE AND COMMIT

TELL YOUR STORY

CONTROL YOUR ENVIRONMENT

EAT MINDFULLY

VISUALIZE YOUR FUTURE

DOCUMENT YOUR JOURNEY

PRACTICE COMPASSION

REDUCE STRESS

DELAY GRATIFICATION

FOCUS ON NUTRIENT-DENSE FOOD

In order to keep you on track with your weight-loss plans, follow these principles and recommit by using motivators such as quotations, photos, books, diaries and recordings. Motivational quotations are located in Appendix E. Here are two of our favorite quotations:

Self-reliance is the only road to true freedom,
and being one's own person is its ultimate reward.
~ PATRICIA SAMPSON

Between stimulus and response there is a space.
In that space is our power to choose our response.
In our response lies our growth and our freedom.
~ VIKTOR E. FRANKL

Appendix A

THE 20 BILLION DOLLAR DIET® GROCERY LIST

Here's a list of some delicious and nutrient-dense foods, the individual tasty elements that comprise a healthy eating pattern. Use the following foods, herbs and spices as a foundation for promoting your health.

Vegetables	Artichoke	Broccoli	Garlic	Peas
	Arugula	Cabbage	Ginger	Potatoes
	Avocado	Carrots	Kale	Red peppers
	Banana peppers	Cauliflower	Mixed greens	Romaine lettuce
	Beets	Celery	Mushrooms	Spinach
	Bell peppers	Corn	Onions	Sweet potatoes
Fruits	Apples	Cherries	Lemons	Peaches
	Avocado	Cranberries	Limes	Pears
	Bananas	Grapes	Mango	Pineapple
	Blackberries	Grapefruit	Melons	Raspberries
	Blueberries	Kiwi fruit	Oranges	Strawberries
Grains	Barley	Bulgur	Oats	Rye
	Brown rice	Cornmeal	Quinoa	Whole wheat
Beans	Black beans	Kidney beans	Pinto beans	Split peas
	Chickpeas (hummus)	Lentils	Red beans	White peas
	Edamame	Soybean products including patties and links and/or tofu		
Dairy	Fat-free milk (or choose almond milk)		Yogurt	Kefir
	Low-fat cheeses (provolone, cheddar, pepper jack, cottage cheese)			
Nuts Seeds	Almonds	Flaxseed meal	Pumpkin seeds	Sunflower seeds
	Chia seeds	Peanuts	Sesame seeds	Walnuts
Herbs Spices	Bay leaf	Cilantro	Nutmeg	Rosemary
	Basil	Cumin	Paprika	Sage
	Black pepper	Fennel	Parsley	Sea salt
	Chai	Garlic	Peppermint	Thyme
	Chili pepper	Ginger	Red pepper	Turmeric
Vinegars Oils	Apple cider vinegar	Balsamic vinegar	Red wine vinegar	Rice vinegar
	Canola oil	Olive oil	Peanut oil	Margarine (zero trans fat)
	Almond butter and/or peanut butter (unsweetened)			

This list is designed to serve as a resource for those who choose to follow a vegetarian plan. Food composition and complete nutrient requirements can be found on the USDA website.

Appendix B

SHOULD I EAT THIS?

When faced with a food choice, try to answer 'yes' to the following questions.

Is this food real with no unpronounceable chemicals and additives?

Is this food plant-based? If not, have I eaten enough plant-based foods to meet my daily needs?

Does this food provide fiber so that I can achieve my 25-gram (minimum) recommended intake*?

Does this food provide protein so that I can achieve my 46-gram Recommended Dietary Allowance*?

Does this food keep me under my 25-gram daily guideline for sugar?

Does this food make a healthy contribution to my daily calorie intake?

*The Recommended Dietary Allowance (RDA) for protein is 0.8 grams of protein per kilogram of body weight for adult men and women. See the ChooseMyPlate and USDA websites for nutritional requirements based on age and gender and for women who are pregnant or lactating.

Appendix C

WHAT DOES 100 CALORIES LOOK LIKE?			
Fruits	**Vegetables**	**Protein**	**Grains**
1 apple	30 spears asparagus	½ cup tuna	¾ cup whole grain (high fiber) cereal*
1 banana	1 head lettuce	1.5 oz hamburger	1 slice whole grain bread*
2 cups watermelon	6 small tomatoes	½ chicken breast	1/3 cup dry oatmeal
1¼ cup blueberries	15 stalks celery	¾ soybean patty*	½ cup (cooked) brown rice
1 peach	4 medium carrots	½ cup black beans	1/6 cup dry quinoa
1 orange	13 cups spinach	½ cup low-fat cottage cheese	1 large slice rye bread*

Appendix D

WOMEN'S DAILY CALORIE REQUIREMENTS FOR WEIGHT MAINTENANCE					
Body weight (lbs)	BMR	sedentary	somewhat active	moderately active	very active
120	1250	1500	1750	1950	2150
130	1300	1550	1800	2000	2250
140	1350	1600	1850	2100	2300
150	1400	1650	1900	2150	2400
160	1450	1700	1950	2200	2500
170	1500	1750	2000	2300	2550
180	1500	1800	2100	2350	2600
190	1550	1850	2150	2400	2700
200	1600	1950	2200	2500	2750
210	1650	2000	2250	2550	2850
220	1700	2050	2350	2600	2900

Women: The table shows the approximate basal metabolic rate (BMR) and calorie requirements for a woman who is 5'6" tall and 49 years of age. Calorie requirements increase with pregnancy and lactation.

Calorie requirements vary with height, age, and activity level. Tables are based on the Harris-Benedict equation. For personalized results, see: http://www.bmi-calculator.net/bmr-calculator/

BMR (Basal Metabolic Rate) is the number of calories you'd burn if you stayed in bed all day. **Sedentary:** Little or no exercise other than housework and/or light gardening. **Somewhat active:** For example, exercising for at least 20 minutes, 1 to 3 days per week. **Moderately active:** For example, exercising for at least 30 to 60 minutes, 3 to 4 days per week. **Very active:** For example, exercising for at least 60 minutes, 5 to 7 days per week.

Adults need at least 2 hours and 30 minutes (150 minutes) of moderate-intensity aerobic activity (i.e., brisk walking) every week and muscle-strengthening activities on 2 or more days a week. See: http://www.cdc.gov/physicalactivity/basics/adults/index.htm

MEN'S DAILY CALORIE REQUIREMENTS FOR WEIGHT MAINTENANCE

Body weight (lbs)	BMR	sedentary	somewhat active	moderately activity	very active
160	1600	1950	2250	2500	2800
170	1700	2000	2300	2600	2900
180	1750	2100	2400	2700	3000
190	1800	2150	2500	2800	3100
200	1850	2250	2550	2900	3200
210	1950	2300	2650	3000	3350
220	2000	2400	2750	3100	3450
230	2050	2450	2850	3200	3550
240	2100	2550	2900	3300	3650
250	2200	2600	3000	3400	3750
260	2250	2700	3100	3500	3850

Men: The table shows the approximate BMR and calorie requirements for a man who is 5'10" tall and 49 years of age.

Calorie requirements vary with height, age, and activity level. Tables are based on the Harris-Benedict equation. For personalized results, see: http://www.bmi-calculator.net/bmr-calculator/

BMR (Basal Metabolic Rate) is the number of calories you'd burn if you stayed in bed all day. **Sedentary**: Little or no exercise other than housework and/or light gardening. **Somewhat active**: For example, exercising for at least 20 minutes, 1 to 3 days per week. **Moderately active**: For example, exercising for at least 30 to 60 minutes, 3 to 4 days per week. **Very active**: For example, exercising for at least 60 minutes, 5 to 7 days per week.

Adults need at least 2 hours and 30 minutes (150 minutes) of moderate-intensity aerobic activity (i.e., brisk walking) every week and muscle-strengthening activities on 2 or more days a week. See: http://www.cdc.gov/physicalactivity/basics/adults/index.htm

Appendix E

Motivational Quotations

The significant problems we have cannot be solved at the same level of thinking with which we created them.
~ ALBERT EINSTEIN

I believe that half the unhappiness in life comes from people being afraid to go straight at things.
~ WILLIAM J. LOCKE

The knowledge that we are responsible for our actions and attitudes does not need to be discouraging, because it also means that we are free to change [our] destiny... We can alter the chemistry provided we have the courage to dissect the elements.
~ ANAÏS NIN

Almost all successful people begin with two beliefs: the future can be better than the present, and I have the power to make it so.
~ DAVID BROOKS, NEW YORK TIMES COLUMNIST

A vision is not just a picture of what could be; it is an appeal to our better selves, a call to become something more.
~ ROSABETH MOSS KANTER

Whether you believe you can do a thing or not, you are right.
~ HENRY FORD

If you can dream it, you can do it.
~ TOM FITZGERALD, WALT DISNEY CORP.

Getting from point A to point Z can be daunting unless you remember that you don't have to get from A to Z. You just have to get from A to B. Breaking big dreams into small steps is the way to move forward.
~ SHERYL SANDBERG, AUTHOR, COO OF FACEBOOK

Thoughts lead on to purposes; purposes go forth in action; actions form habits; habits decide character; and character fixes our destiny.
~TYRON EDWARDS

To learn new habits is everything, for it is to reach the substance of life. Life is but a tissue of habits.
~ HENRI FREDERIC AMIEL

We can use decision-making to choose the habits we want to form, use willpower to get the habit started, then - and this is the best part - we can allow the extraordinary power of habit to take over. At that point, we're free from the need to decide and the need to use willpower.
~ GRETCHEN RUBIN

Knowing is not enough; we must apply. Willing is not enough; we must do.
~ JOHANN WOLFGANG VON GOETHE

*You have a choice. Mindsets are just beliefs. They're powerful
beliefs, but they're just something in your mind,
and you can change your mind.*
~ CAROL S. DWECK, FROM *MINDSET: THE NEW
PSYCHOLOGY OF SUCCESS*

*Feelings come and go like clouds in a windy sky. Conscious
breathing is my anchor.*
~ THICH NHAT HANH, FROM *STEPPING INTO FREEDOM:
RULES OF MONASTIC PRACTICE FOR NOVICES*

*With self-kindness, we soothe and calm our troubled minds.
We make a peace offering of warmth, gentleness and
sympathy from ourselves to ourselves,
so that true healing can occur.*
~ KRISTIN NEFF, FROM *SELF-COMPASSION: THE PROVEN
POWER OF BEING KIND TO YOURSELF.*

*Between stimulus and response there is a space. In that space is
our power to choose our response. In our response
lies our growth and our freedom.*
~ VIKTOR E. FRANKL

*I believe that anyone can conquer fear by doing the things he
fears to do, provided he keeps doing them until he gets a record
of successful experiences behind him.*
~ ELEANOR ROOSEVELT

*Self-reliance is the only road to true freedom, and being one's
own person is its ultimate reward.*
~ PATRICIA SAMPSON

He who controls others may be powerful, but he who has
mastered himself is mightier still.
~ LAO TZU

True happiness involves the full use of one's power and talents.
~ JOHN W. GARDNER

Everybody in the world is seeking happiness—and there is
one sure way to find it. That is by controlling your thoughts.
Happiness doesn't depend on outward conditions.
It depends on inner conditions.
~ DALE CARNEGIE, FROM *HOW TO WIN*
FRIENDS AND INFLUENCE PEOPLE

Additional Reading

Albers, Susan, PSY.D. (2009). *50 ways to soothe yourself without food*. Oakland, CA: New Harbinger Publications, Inc. Website: http://eatingmindfully.com/

Albers, Susan, PSY.D. (2011). *"But I deserve this chocolate!" The 50 most common diet-derailing excuses and how to outwit them."* Oakland, CA: New Harbinger Publications, Inc. Website: http://eatingmindfully.com/

Burns, David D., M.D. (1980). *Feeling good: The new mood therapy*. New York: Avon Books. Website: http://feelinggood.com

Cameron, Julia. (2007). *The writing diet: Write yourself right-size*. New York: Penguin.

Cohen, Deborah A., M.D. (2014). *A big fat crisis: The hidden forces behind the obesity epidemic – and how we can end it*. New York: Nation Books. Website: http://www.abigfatcrisis.com/

Duhigg, Charles (2012). *The power of habit: Why we do what we do in life and business*. New York: Random House. Website: http://charlesduhigg.com/

Dweck, Carol S., Ph.D. (2006). *Mindset: The new psychology of success*. New York: Ballantine Books. Website: http://mindsetonline.com/

Kabat-Zinn, Jon (1994). *Wherever you go, there you are*. New York: MJF Books. Website: http://www.mindfulnesscds.com/

Kessler, David A., M.D. (2009). *The end of overeating: Taking control of the insatiable American appetite*. New York: Rodale Inc.

Lustig, Robert H., M.D. (2013). *Fat chance: Beating the odds against sugar, processed food, obesity, and disease*. New York: Hudson Street Press.

McGonigal, Kelly, Ph.D. (2012). *The willpower instinct: How self-control works, why it matters, and what you can do to get more of it.* New York: Avery (The Penguin Group). Website: http://kellymcgonigal.com/

Mischel, Walter, Ph.D. (2014). *The marshmallow test: Mastering self-control.* New York: Little, Brown and Company.

Neff, Kristin, Ph.D. (2011). *Self-Compassion: The proven power of being kind to yourself.* New York: HarperCollins. Website: http://self-compassion.org/

Pollan, Michael (2014). *Cooked.* New York: Penguin. Website: http://michaelpollan.com/

Otto, Michael, Ph.D., and Smits, Jasper, Ph.D. (2010). *Exercise for mood and anxiety: Proven strategies for overcoming depression and enhancing well-being.* New York: Oxford University Press.

Sonnenburg, Justin and Erica, Ph.Ds. (2015). *The good gut: Taking control of your weight, your mood, and your long-term health.* New York: Penguin.

Wansink, Brian, Ph.D. (2006). *Mindless eating: Why we eat more than we think.* New York: Bantam Books. Website: http://mindlesseating.org/

Wansink, Brian, Ph.D. (2014). *Slim by Design: Mindless eating solutions for everyday life.* New York: HarperCollins. Website: http://mindlesseating.org/

Weil, Andrew, M.D. (1995). *Natural health, natural medicine.* Boston/New York: Houghton Mifflin. Website: http://www.drweil.com/

Williamson, Marianne (2010). *A course in weight loss: 21 lessons for surrendering your weight forever.* CA: Hay House. Website: http://marianne.com/

Scientific Citations

The scientific citations and articles mentioned in the chapters are indexed to key phrases in the text.

INTRODUCTION

Americans spend more than $20 billion on weight loss:
(1) ABC News. (2012). 100 million dieters, $20 billion: The weight-loss industry by the numbers. May 8, 2012. Retrieved from <http://abcnews.go.com/Health/100-million-dieters-20-billion-weight-loss-industry/story?id=16297197 >
(2) *The numbers are even higher if diet soft drinks are included*: PRWEB. (2012). U.S. Weight loss market forecast to hit $66 billion in 2013. Dec 31, 2012. Retrieved from <http://www.prweb.com/releases/2012/12/prweb10278281.htm>
(3) US News & World Report. The heavy price of losing weight. (2013). Retrieved from <http://money.usnews.com/money/personal-finance/articles/2013/01/02/the-heavy-price-of-losing-weight >
(4) *The diet industry in Europe and United States has an annual turnover in excess of $150 billion*: Dulloo, A. G., & Montani, J. P. (2015). Pathways from dieting to weight regain, to obesity and to the metabolic syndrome: An overview. *Obesity Reviews, 16*(S1), 1-6.
(5) *The average cost per kilogram of weight lost ranges from $155 to $546*: Finkelstein, E. A., & Kruger, E. (2014). Meta-and cost-effectiveness analysis of commercial weight loss strategies. *Obesity, 22*(9), 1942-1951.

The obesity rate is higher than ever:
(1) *Gallup poll*: Levy, J. (2015). U.S. obesity rate inches up to 27.7% in 2014. Jan. 26, 2015. Retrieved from <http://www.gallup.com/poll/181271/obesity-rate-inches-2014.aspx>
(2) Blazek, N. (2011). Half of Americans expected to be obese in 2030. *The Clinical Advisor*, Aug. 26, 2011. Retrieved from <http://www.clinicaladvisor.com/half-of-americans-expected-to-be-obese-in-2030/article/210605/>

(3) Wang, Y. C., McPherson, K., Marsh, T., Gortmaker, S. L., & Brown, M. (2011). Health and economic burden of the projected obesity trends in the USA and the UK. *The Lancet, 378*(9793), 815-825.

The average dieter gained almost five pounds in a year: Post, R. E., Johnson, S. P., Wright, R. U., & Mainous 3rd, A. G. (2014). Comparison of traditional and nontraditional weight loss methods: An analysis of the National Health and Nutrition Examination Survey. *Southern Medical Journal, 107*(7), 410-415.

America is on a $20 billion diet that isn't working:
(1) *One third to two thirds of dieters regain more weight than they lost on their diets:* Mann, T., Tomiyama, A. J., Westling, E., Lew, A. M., Samuels, B., & Chatman, J. (2007). Medicare's search for effective obesity treatments: Diets are not the answer. *American Psychologist, 62*(3), 220.
(2) *The fad diet industry derives billions of dollars from a nation that is not getting healthier:* Pagoto, S. L., & Appelhans, B. M. (2013). A call for an end to the diet debates. *JAMA, 310*(7), 687-688.
(3) *Liquid diets, nonprescription diet pills, and popular diets are not successful:* Nicklas, J. M., Huskey, K. W., Davis, R. B., & Wee, C. C. (2012). Successful weight loss among obese US adults. *American Journal of Preventive Medicine, 42*(5), 481-485.
(4) *There is little difference in weight loss on popular diets:* Atallah, R., Filion, K. B., Wakil, S. M., Genest, J., Joseph, L., Poirier, P., ... & Eisenberg, M. J. (2014). Long-term effects of 4 popular diets on weight loss and cardio-vascular risk factors: A systematic review of randomized controlled trials. *Circulation: Cardiovascular Quality and Outcomes, 7*(6), 815-827.
(5) *Herbal supplements are ineffective:* Esteghamati, A., Mazaheri, T., Rad, M. V., & Noshad, S. (2015). Complementary and alternative medicine for the treatment of obesity: A critical review. *International Journal of Endocrinology and Metabolism, 13*(2).
(6) *Herbal supplements are often dangerous:* Stickel, F., & Shouval, D. (2015). Hepatotoxicity of herbal and dietary supplements: An update. *Archives of Toxicology, 89*(6), 851-865.

(7) *Medically supervised very-low-calorie diet programs are associated with high costs, high attrition rates, and a high probability of regaining 50% or more of lost weight in 1 to 2 years*: Tsai, A. G., and Wadden, T. A. (2005). Systematic review: An evaluation of major commercial weight loss programs in the United States. *Annals of Internal Medicine, 142*(1), 56-66.

Oprah and medically-supervised diet:
(1) *Most of the participants who completed the Optifast program regained the weight within a year or two:* Brody, J.E. Diet that made Oprah Winfrey slim demands discipline, specialists say. *The New York Times*, Nov 24, 1988.
(2) Winfrey, O. How did I let this happen again? *O, The Oprah Magazine*, Jan 2009.

When I took complete ownership, I was successful: *Behavior change is more likely to occur if it is autonomously motivated*:
(1) Williams, G. C., Grow, V. M., Freedman, Z. R., Ryan, R. M., & Deci, E. L. (1996). Motivational predictors of weight loss and weight-loss maintenance. *Journal of Personality and Social Psychology, 70*(1), 115.
(2) Verstuyf, J., Patrick, H., Vansteenkiste, M., & Teixeira, P. J. (2012). Motivational dynamics of eating regulation: A self-determination theory perspective. *International Journal of Behavioral Nutrition and Physical Activity, 9*(1), 1-16.
(3) De Ridder, D. T., & De Wit, J. B. (2006). Self-regulation in health behavior: Concepts, theories, and central issues. *Self-regulation in Health Behavior*, edited by D. de Ridder and J. de Wit (UK: John Wiley & Sons Ltd.)

CHAPTER 1. BELIEVE AND COMMIT
Power in making a commitment: *If individuals fully endorse weight loss goals, and feel competent and autonomous about reaching them, they are more likely to succeed*:
Teixeira, P. J., Silva, M. N., Mata, J., Palmeira, A. L., & Markland, D. (2012). Motivation, self-determination, and long-term weight control. *Int J Behav Nutr Phys Act, 9*(1), 22.

An important aspect of commitment is weighing the pros and cons: Prochaska, J. O., DiClemente, C. C., and Norcross, J. C. (1992). In search of how people change: Applications to addictive behaviors. *American Psychologist, 47*(9), 1102.

Self-efficacy theory: Bandura, A. (1977). Self-efficacy: Toward a unifying theory of behavioral change. *Psychological Review, 84*(2), 191.

Self-efficacy and weight loss:
(1) *Participants who had higher self-efficacy lost more weight*: Shin, H., Shin, J., Liu, P. Y., Dutton, G. R., Abood, D. A., & Ilich, J. Z. (2011). Self-efficacy improves weight loss in overweight/obese postmenopausal women during a 6-month weight loss intervention. *Nutrition Research, 31*(11), 822-828.
(2) Kreausukon, P., Gellert, P., Lippke, S., & Schwarzer, R. (2012). Planning and self-efficacy can increase fruit and vegetable consumption: A randomized controlled trial. *Journal of Behavioral Medicine, 35*(4), 443-451.
(3) Cochrane, G. (2008). Role for a sense of self-worth in weight-loss treatments: Helping patients develop self-efficacy. *Canadian Family Physician, 54*(4), 543-547.
(4) Annesi, J. J., & Gorjala, S. (2010). Relations of self-regulation and self-efficacy for exercise and eating and BMI change: A field investigation. *Biopsychosoc Med, 4*(10), 269-278.
(5) *Self-affirmation as a tool*: Epton, T., and Harris, P. R. (2008). Self-affirmation promotes health behavior change. *Health Psychology, 27*(6), 746.

Whether you believe you can do a thing or not, you are right: *The attribution is discussed at Quote Investigator*: Retrieved from < http://quoteinvestigator.com/2015/02/03/you-can/>

Willpower - reason for failure?
(1) American Psychological Association. (2012). What Americans think of willpower: A survey of perceptions of willpower and its role in achieving lifestyle and behavior-change goals. 2011 Stress in America™ survey, copyright 2012, American Psychological Association.

(2) Former FDA commissioner Dr. David Kessler says: "Conditioned hypereating is a biological challenge, not a character flaw. Recovery is impossible until we stop viewing overeating as an absence of willpower." p. 206 in: Kessler, David A., M.D. (2009). *The end of overeating: taking control of the insatiable American appetite*. New York: Rodale Inc.

(3) Dr. Brian Wansink says: "One sentence summarizes twenty-five years of my research: Becoming slim by design works better than trying to become slim by willpower. That is, it's easier to change your eating environment than to change your mind." p. 6 in: Wansink, Brian Ph.D. (2014). *Slim by Design: Mindless eating solutions for everyday life*. New York: HarperCollins.

(4) Implicit beliefs about willpower can become either an obstacle or an aid for dieters. A perceived lack of willpower leads to relinquishing of personal autonomy: Beruchashvili, M., & Moisio, R. (2013). Is planning an aid or an obstacle? Examining the role of consumers' lay theories in weight loss. *Journal of Consumer Affairs*, *47*(3), 404-431.

Willpower may not be limited after all: Carter, E. C., Kofler, L. M., Forster, D. E., & McCullough, M. E. (2015). A series of meta-analytic tests of the depletion effect: Self-control does not seem to rely on a limited resource. *Journal of Experimental Psychology (General)*, *144*(4), 796-815.

Beliefs affect outcomes (Dweck et al.):
(1) Job, V., Dweck, C. S., & Walton, G. M. (2010). Ego depletion—Is it all in your head? Implicit theories about willpower affect self-regulation. *Psychological Science 21*(11), 1686-1693.
(2) Job, V., Walton, G. M., Bernecker, K., & Dweck, C. S. (2013). Beliefs about willpower determine the impact of glucose on self-control. *Proceedings of the National Academy of Sciences*, *110*(37), 14837-14842.
(3) Job, V., Walton, G. M., Bernecker, K., & Dweck, C. S. (2015). Implicit theories about willpower predict self-regulation and grades in everyday life. *Journal of Personality and Social Psychology*, *108*(4), 637.
(4) Walton, G., & Dweck, C. Willpower: It's in your head. *The New York Times*, Nov 26, 2011.

A simple implementation intention improves outcomes: Implementation intentions always specify a cue (such as, "*if* I start a new problem"). The response ("*then* I will….") proceeds automatically when the cue is encountered. Participants who stated "If I start a new problem, then I will tell myself: I can solve it') solved more problems: Bayer, U. C., & Gollwitzer, P. M. (2007). Boosting scholastic test scores by willpower: The role of implementation intentions. *Self and Identity, 6*(1), 1-19.

View the situation as a challenge with a desirable goal (to prove that you have willpower):
(1) *Reframing of rewards can promote self-control while avoiding the need for additional willpower*: Magen, E., Kim, B., Dweck, C. S., Gross, J. J., & McClure, S. M. (2014). Behavioral and neural correlates of increased self-control in the absence of increased willpower. *Proceedings of the National Academy of Sciences, 111*(27), 9786-9791.
(2) *Reframing temptation as a test of willpower*: Magen, E., & Gross, J. J. (2007). Harnessing the need for immediate gratification: Cognitive reconstrual modulates the reward value of temptations. *Emotion, 7*(2), 415.
(3) *Participants who understood the task as a test of willpower performed better*: Leroy, V., Grégoire, J., Magen, E., Gross, J. J., & Mikolajczak, M. (2012). Lead me not into temptation: Using cognitive reappraisal to reduce goal-inconsistent behavior. *PLoS One, 7*(7), e39493-e39493.

Strategies that reduce the need for willpower are most effective:
(1) *Perhaps the most important self-control tactic is to avoid the types of situations that induce intense visceral responses*: Loewenstein, G. (2000). Willpower: A decision-theorist's perspective. *Law and Philosophy, 19*(1), 51-76.
(2)Hofmann, W., Baumeister, R. F., Förster, G., & Vohs, K. D. (2012). Everyday temptations: An experience sampling study of desire, conflict, and self-control. *Journal of Personality and Social Psychology, 102*(6), 1318.
(3) de Ridder, D. T., Lensvelt-Mulders, G., Finkenauer, C., Stok, F. M., & Baumeister, R. F. (2012). Taking stock of self-control: A meta-analysis of how trait self-control relates to a wide range of behaviors. *Personality and Social Psychology Review, 16*(1), 76-99.

(4) Ent, M. R., Baumeister, R. F., & Tice, D. M. (2015). Trait self-control and the avoidance of temptation. *Personality and Individual Differences, 74*, 12-15. *For commentary see*: Lukits, A. The secret to resisting temptation: People who excel at resisting temptation deliberately avoid tempting situations, says a study. *The Wall Street Journal*, Nov 24, 2014.

(5) *Temptation resistance strategies ("hot state" strategies) rely on willpower. By contrast, temptation prevention strategies are implemented in a "cold state" with the aim of avoiding future temptations*: Appelhans, B. M., French, S. A., Pagoto, S. L., & Sherwood, N. E. (2016). Managing temptation in obesity treatment: A neurobehavioral model of intervention strategies. Appetite, 96, 268-279.

(6) *People with high self-control use their self-control less frequently as a result of having established effective habits or routines, rather than being more successful in resisting single temptations*: Adriaanse, M. A., Kroese, F. M., Gillebaart, M., & De Ridder, D. T. (2014). Effortless inhibition: Habit mediates the relation between self-control and unhealthy snack consumption. *Frontiers in Psychology, 5*, 444.

(7) *Individuals with self-control use less effort by relying on beneficial habits*: Galla, B. M., & Duckworth, A. L. (2015). More than resisting temptation: Beneficial habits mediate the relationship between self-control and positive life outcomes. *Journal of Personality and Social Psychology 109*(3), 508.

Believing in your abilities shifts neural responses: *"Believing that you can accomplish what you want to accomplish is one of the most important ingredients – perhaps the most important ingredient – in the recipe for success."* Maddux, J. E. (2009). Self-efficacy: The power of believing you can. *The Oxford Handbook of Positive Psychology* (2nd ed.), edited by Shane J. Lopez and C.R. Snyder.

Carrying on in the face of challenges or setbacks impels change:
(1) *Self-control can be strengthened through practice*: Muraven, M. (2010). Building self-control strength: Practicing self-control leads to improved self-control performance. *Journal of Experimental Social Psychology, 46*(2), 465-468.

(2) Berkman, E. T., Graham, A. M., & Fisher, P. A. (2012). Training self-control: A domain-general translational neuroscience approach. *Child Development Perspectives*, *6*(4), 374-384.

(3) *Successful dieters had a greater activation in the dorsal prefrontal cortex, dorsal striatum and anterior cerebellar lobe as compared to non-dieters*: DelParigi, A., Chen, K., Salbe, A. D., Hill, J. O., Wing, R. R., Reiman, E. M., & Tataranni, P. A. (2007). Successful dieters have increased neural activity in cortical areas involved in the control of behavior. *International Journal of Obesity*, *31*(3), 440-448.

CHAPTER 2. TELL YOUR STORY

I noticed that models and actresses were extremely thin: Mass media promote a thin body ideal that elicits body dissatisfaction:

(1) Groesz, L. M., Levine, M. P., & Murnen, S. K. (2002). The effect of experimental presentation of thin media images on body satisfaction: A meta-analytic review. *International Journal of Eating Disorders*, *31*(1), 1-16.

(2) Neumark-Sztainer, D., Wall, M., Story, M., & Sherwood, N. E. (2009). Five-year longitudinal predictive factors for disordered eating in a population-based sample of overweight adolescents: Implications for prevention and treatment. *International Journal of Eating Disorders*, *42*(7), 664-672.

(3) Monro, F., & Huon, G. (2005). Media-portrayed idealized images, body shame, and appearance anxiety. *International Journal of Eating Disorders*, *38*(1), 85-90.

(4) van den Berg, P., Neumark-Sztainer, D., Hannan, P. J., & Haines, J. (2007). Is dieting advice from magazines helpful or harmful? Five-year associations with weight-control behaviors and psychological outcomes in adolescents. *Pediatrics*, *119*(1), e30-e37.

Skipping breakfast, a lifetime of weight struggles:

(1) Niemeier, H. M., Raynor, H. A., Lloyd-Richardson, E. E., Rogers, M. L., & Wing, R. R. (2006). Fast food consumption and breakfast skipping: Predictors of weight gain from adolescence to adulthood in a nationally representative sample. *Journal of Adolescent Health*, *39*(6), 842-849.

(2) *Skipping meals predicted increases in BMI*: Neumark-Sztainer, D., Wall, M., Story, M., & Standish, A. R. (2012). Dieting and unhealthy weight control behaviors during adolescence: associations with 10-year changes in body mass index. *Journal of Adolescent Health*, *50*(1), 80-86.

(3) *Importance of a breakfast containing protein*: Leidy, H. J., Ortinau, L. C., Douglas, S. M., & Hoertel, H. A. (2013). Beneficial effects of a higher-protein breakfast on the appetitive, hormonal, and neural signals controlling energy intake regulation in overweight/obese, breakfast-skipping, late-adolescent girls. *The American Journal of Clinical Nutrition*, *97*(4), 677-688.

(4) *Eating breakfast reduced cravings*: Hoertel, H. A., Will, M. J., & Leidy, H. J. (2014). A randomized crossover, pilot study examining the effects of a normal protein vs. high protein breakfast on food cravings and reward signals in overweight/obese "breakfast skipping", late-adolescent girls. *Nutrition Journal*, *13*(1), 80.

(5) *Adolescent females with more frequent breakfast and dinner consumption were protected against becoming overweight*: Quick, V., Wall, M., Larson, N., Haines, J., & Neumark-Sztainer, D. (2013). Personal, behavioral and socio-environmental predictors of overweight incidence in young adults: 10-yr longitudinal findings. *Int J Behav Nutr Phys Act*, *10*(1), 37.

Food restriction can precipitate binge eating and obesity:

(1) *Food restriction intensifies the desire for sugar and fat*: Cameron, J. D., Goldfield, G. S., Finlayson, G., Blundell, J. E., & Doucet, É. (2014). Fasting for 24 hours heightens reward from food and food-related cues. *PLoS One*, *9*(1), e85970.

(2) Goldstone, A. P., Prechtl de Hernandez, C. G., Beaver, J. D., Muhammed, K., Croese, C., Bell, G., ... & Bell, J. D. (2009). Fasting biases brain reward systems towards high-calorie foods. *European Journal of Neuroscience*, *30*(8), 1625-1635.

(3) Macpherson-Sánchez, A. E. (2015). Integrating fundamental concepts of obesity and eating disorders: implications for the obesity epidemic. *American Journal of Public Health*, *105*(4), e71-85.

(4) Hagan, M. M., Tomaka, J., & Moss, D. E. (2000). Relation of dieting in college and high school students to symptoms associated with semi-starvation. *Journal of Health Psychology*, *5*(1), 7-15.

Neural circuit that controls compulsive sugar consumption:
(1) Nieh, E. H., Matthews, G. A., Allsop, S. A., Presbrey, K. N., Leppla, C. A., Wichmann, R., ... & Tye, K. M. (2015). Decoding neural circuits that control compulsive sucrose seeking. *Cell, 160*(3), 528-541.
(2) Cell Press. Researchers discover brain circuit that controls compulsive overeating and sugar addiction. Jan. 29, 2015. Retrieved from <http://www.eurekalert.org/pub_releases/2015-01/cp-rdb012315.php>
(3) Denis, R. G., Joly-Amado, A., Webber, E., Langlet, F., Schaeffer, M., Padilla, S. L., ... & Martinez, S. (2015). Palatability can drive feeding independent of AgRP neurons. *Cell Metabolism, 22*(4), 646-657.

Animals can be turned into binge eaters:
(1) Corwin, R. L., Avena, N. M., & Boggiano, M. M. (2011). Feeding and reward: Perspectives from three rat models of binge eating. *Physiology & Behavior, 104*(1), 87-97.
(2) *Rats exhibited binge eating on a solution of corn oil, heavy cream and sugar (similar to ice cream):* Lardeux, S., Kim, J. J., & Nicola, S. M. (2013). Intermittent access to sweet high-fat liquid induces increased palatability and motivation to consume in a rat model of binge consumption. *Physiology & Behavior, 114*, 21-31.
(3) *As evidence of addiction, binge-eating animals will tolerate punishment in order to obtain chocolate:* Oswald, K. D., Murdaugh, D. L., King, V. L., & Boggiano, M. M. (2011). Motivation for palatable food despite consequences in an animal model of binge eating. *International Journal of Eating Disorders, 44*(3), 203-211.

Adaptations in the brain are similar to changes seen with addictive drugs:
(1) Rada, P., Avena, N. M., & Hoebel, B. G. (2005). Daily bingeing on sugar repeatedly releases dopamine in the accumbens shell. *Neuroscience, 134*(3), 737-744.
(2) Hoebel, B. (2009). Sugar addiction: Bingeing, withdrawal, and craving. *Obesity and Food Addiction Summit: The Obesity Epidemic Connection*. Retrieved from <http://www.foodaddictionsummit.org/presenters-hoebel.htm>

(3) Bartoshuk, L. (2009). Addicted to food: An interview with Bart Hoebel. *APS Observer 22*(9).

Sugar is a big part of the problem:
(1) Avena, N.M., Rada, P., & Hoebel, B.G. (2008). Evidence of sugar addiction: Behavioral and neurochemical effects of intermittent, excessive sugar intake. *Neuroscience & Biobehavioral Reviews, 32*(1), 20-39.
(2) Avena, N. M., Rada, P., & Hoebel, B. G. (2009). Sugar and fat bingeing have notable differences in addictive-like behavior. *The Journal of Nutrition, 139*(3), 623-628.
(3) *High-sugar foods may circumvent satiety mechanisms:* Mitra, A., Gosnell, B. A., Schiöth, H. B., Grace, M. K., Klockars, A., Olszewski, P. K., & Levine, A. S. (2010). Chronic sugar intake dampens feeding-related activity of neurons synthesizing a satiety mediator, oxytocin. *Peptides, 31*(7), 1346-1352.

Most of which was probably water loss:
(1) *Extreme diets initially induce dehydration:* Zamora Navarro, S. Z., & Pérez-Llamas, F. (2013). Errors and myths in feeding and nutrition: Impact on the problems of obesity. *Nutr Hosp, 28*(Supl 5), 81-88.
(2) *Lean mass is lost:* Beavers, K. M., Lyles, M. F., Davis, C. C., Wang, X., Beavers, D. P., & Nicklas, B. J. (2011). Is lost lean mass from intentional weight loss recovered during weight regain in postmenopausal women? *The American Journal of Clinical Nutrition, 94*(3), 767-774.

Even if binge eating occurs less frequently, it is a problem for many individuals:
(1) Greeno, C. G., Wing, R. R., & Shiffman, S. (2000). Binge antecedents in obese women with and without binge eating disorder. *Journal of Consulting and Clinical Psychology, 68*(1), 95.
(2) *In one survey, almost half of the women said they snacked in secret, and more than a quarter confessed to binge eating:* Press Association. Women own up to guilt over eating habits. The Guardian, Jan 19, 2013.

(3) *When Americans were asked to recall the last time they overate to the point of regret, 83% had done it within the past 10 days:* Wansink, B., & Chandon, P. (2014). Slim by design: Redirecting the accidental drivers of mindless overeating. *Journal of Consumer Psychology, 24*(3), 413-431.

Official diagnostic criteria for binge-eating disorder: American Psychiatric Association. (2013). Feeding and Eating Disorders. *Diagnostic and Statistical Manual of Mental Disorders*, 5th ed. Washington, DC: American Psychiatric Association.

There is a spectrum of overeating, from mild to severe:
(1) Davis, C. (2013). From passive overeating to 'food addiction': A spectrum of compulsion and severity. *ISRN Obesity, 2013*:435027.
(2) Werdell, P. From the front lines: A clinical approach to food and addiction. *Food and Addiction: A Comprehensive Handbook.* (Oxford, UK: Oxford University Press, 2012.)

Overeating when faced with stress or challenges:
(1) Yau, Y. H., & Potenza, M. N. (2013). Stress and eating behaviors. *Minerva Endocrinologica, 38*(3), 255.
(2) Groesz, L. M., McCoy, S., Carl, J., Saslow, L., Stewart, J., Adler, N., ... & Epel, E. (2012). What is eating you? Stress and the drive to eat. *Appetite, 58*(2), 717-721.
(3) Jastreboff, A. M., Sinha, R., Lacadie, C., Small, D. M., Sherwin, R. S., & Potenza, M. N. (2013). Neural correlates of stress-and food cue–induced food craving in obesity: Association with insulin levels. *Diabetes Care, 36*(2), 394-402.
(4) *The late afternoon on weekdays is a common time of day for stress-induced eating.* Huh, J., Shiyko, M., Keller, S., Dunton, G., & Schembre, S. M. (2015). The time-varying association between perceived stress and hunger within and between days. *Appetite, 89*, 145-151.
(5) Schellekens H., Finger, B. C., Dinan, T. G., & Cryan, J. F. (2012). Ghrelin signaling and obesity: At the interface of stress, mood and food reward. *Pharmacology and Therapeutics, 135*(3), 316-326.

Like many single women, I was not taking care of myself:
(1) *Mothers in the "sandwich generation," ages 35-54, feel more stress than any other age group as they balance the acts of caring for growing children and their aging parents*: American Psychological Association. (2007). Sandwich generation moms feeling the squeeze. Retrieved from <http://www.apa.org/helpcenter/sandwich-generation.aspx>
(2) Epel, E., Lapidus, R., McEwen, B., & Brownell, K. (2001). Stress may add bite to appetite in women: A laboratory study of stress-induced cortisol and eating behavior. *Psychoneuroendocrinology*, *26*(1), 37-49.
(3) Tomiyama, A. J., Dallman, M. F., & Epel, E. S. (2011). Comfort food is comforting to those most stressed: Evidence of the chronic stress response network in high stress women. *Psychoneuroendocrinology*, *36*(10), 1513-1519.

Compulsive overeating is similar to substance abuse:
(1) Dill, B., and Holton, R. (2014). The addict in us all. *Frontiers in Psychiatry*, *5*, 139.
(2) Alsiö, J., Olszewski, P. K., Levine, A. S., & Schiöth, H. B. (2012). Feedforward mechanisms: Addiction-like behavioral and molecular adaptations in overeating. *Frontiers in Neuroendocrinology*, *33*(2), 127-139.
(3) Vanbuskirk, K. A., & Potenza, M. N. (2010). The treatment of obesity and its co-occurrence with substance use disorders. *Journal of Addiction Medicine*, *4*(1), 1.
(4) Davis, C. (2014). Evolutionary and neuropsychological perspectives on addictive behaviors and addictive substances: Relevance to the 'food addiction' construct. *Substance Abuse and Rehabilitation*, *5*, 129.

Addictive eating behavior, Yale Food Addiction Scale:
The American Psychiatric Association has not yet recognized food addiction as either an eating disorder or a substance abuse disorder. Experts are debating the subject. The use of the word "addiction" to represent any form of overeating has implications for social policy, medicine, and insurance:
(1) Pursey, K. M., Stanwell, P., Gearhardt, A. N., Collins, C. E., & Burrows, T. L. (2014). The prevalence of food addiction as assessed by the Yale Food Addiction Scale: A systematic review. *Nutrients*, *6*(10), 4552-4590.

(2) Meule, A., & Gearhardt, A. N. (2014). Five years of the Yale Food Addiction Scale: Taking stock and moving forward. *Current Addiction Reports, 1*(3), 193-205.

(3) Allen, P. J., Batra, P., Geiger, B. M., Wommack, T., Gilhooly, C., & Pothos, E. N. (2012). Rationale and consequences of reclassifying obesity as an addictive disorder: Neurobiology, food environment and social policy perspectives. *Physiology and Behavior, 107*(1), 126-137.

(4) Taylor, V. H., Curtis, C. M., & Davis, C. (2010). The obesity epidemic: The role of addiction. *Canadian Medical Association Journal, 182*(4), 327-328.

Binge Eating Disorder - high scores on the Yale Food Addiction Scale:
Gearhardt, A. N., White, M. A., & Potenza, M. N. (2011). Binge eating disorder and food addiction. *Current Drug Abuse Reviews, 4*(3), 201.

Feelings of guilt and shame are common and counter-productive:
(1) Chao, Y. H., Yang, C. C., & Chiou, W. B. (2012). Food as ego-protective remedy for people experiencing shame: Experimental evidence for a new perspective on weight-related shame. *Appetite, 59*(2), 570-575.

(2) *An episode of overeating might make us more susceptible to binge eating in the future, in a self-perpetuating spiral*: Polivy, J., & Herman, C. P. (1985). Dieting and binging: A causal analysis. *American Psychologist, 40*(2), 193.

(3) Adam, T. C., & Epel, E. S. (2007). Stress, eating and the reward system. *Physiology & Behavior, 91*(4), 449-458.

Animals – which do not have moral failings – also overeat under conditions that simulate obesogenic environments:
(1) *Eating a Western-style diet contributed to a loss of internal control over appetitive behavior relative to external cues*: Sample, C. H., Martin, A. A., Jones, S., Hargrave, S. L., & Davidson, T. L. (2015). Western-style diet impairs stimulus control by food deprivation state cues: Implications for obesogenic environments. Appetite, 93, 13-23.

(2) *Female rats with a history of intermittent food restriction show binge-like palatable food consumption after 15 min exposure to the sight of the palatable food*: Di Bonaventura, M. V. M., Ciccocioppo, R., Romano, A., Bossert, J. M., Rice, K. C., Ubaldi, M., ... & Cifani, C. (2014). Role of bed nucleus of the stria terminalis corticotrophin-releasing factor receptors in frustration stress-induced binge-like palatable food consumption in female rats with a history of food restriction. The Journal of Neuroscience, 34(34), 11316-11324.

(3) Bocarsly, M. E., & Avena, N. M. (2013). Animal models of binge eating palatable foods: Emergence of addiction-like behaviors and brain changes in the rat. *Animal Models of Eating Disorders*, 179-191.

The relationship between diet and exercise:

(1) *Exercise reduces the intake of hyperpalatable foods in an animal model*: Liang N. C., Bello, N. T., & Moran, T. H. (2015). Wheel running reduces high-fat diet intake, preference and mu-opioid agonist stimulated intake. *Behavioural Brain Research*, *284*, 1-10.

(2) *Exercise reduces urges for sugary snacks*: Ledochowski, L., Ruedl, G., Taylor, A. H., & Kopp, M. (2015). Acute effects of brisk walking on sugary snack cravings in overweight people, affect and responses to a manipulated stress situation and to a sugary snack cue: A crossover study. *PloS One*, *10*(3), e0119278.

(3) *Exercise influences our responses to hyperpalatable food*: Evero, N., Hackett, L. C., Clark, R. D., Phelan, S., & Hagobian, T. A. (2012). Aerobic exercise reduces neuronal responses in food reward brain regions. *Journal of Applied Physiology*, *112*(9), 1612-1619.

(4) *Exercise reduces cravings*: Oh, H., & Taylor, A. H. (2013). A brisk walk, compared with being sedentary, reduces attentional bias and chocolate cravings among regular chocolate eaters with different body mass. *Appetite*, *71*, 144-149.

(5) Cornier, M. A., Melanson, E. L., Salzberg, A. K., Bechtell, J. L., & Tregellas, J. R. (2012). The effects of exercise on the neuronal response to food cues. *Physiology & Behavior*, *105*(4), 1028-1034.

The relationship between exercise, stress and fatigue:
(1) Stults-Kolehmainen M. A., & Sinha, R. (2014). The effects of stress on physical activity and exercise. *Sports Medicine, 44*(1), 81-121.
(2) *Physical activity (20 minutes or more at least once a week) reduced the risk of fatigue in nurse's aides.* Eriksen, W., & Bruusgaard, D. (2004). Do physical leisure time activities prevent fatigue? A 15-month prospective study of nurses' aides. *British Journal of Sports Medicine, 38*(3), 331-336.

Justifications are commonly used by people who overeat:
(1) Taylor, C., Webb, T. L., & Sheeran, P. (2014). I deserve a treat!: Justifications for indulgence undermine the translation of intentions into action. *British Journal of Social Psychology, 53*(3), 501-520.
(2) Huberts, J. C. D. W., Evers, C., & De Ridder, D. T. (2014). Because I am worth it: A theoretical framework and empirical review of a justification-based account of self-regulation failure. *Personality and Social Psychology Review, 18*(2), 119-138.
(3) de Witt Huberts, J., Evers, C., & de Ridder, D. (2014). Thinking before sinning: reasoning processes in hedonic consumption. *Frontiers in Psychology, 5,* 1268.
(4) *People often justify indulgences when they think that sufficient progress toward their goal has been made*: Hofmann, W., & Van Dillen, L. (2012). Desire: The new hot spot in self-control research. *Current Directions in Psychological Science, 21*(5), 317-322.

We protect our egos by defending our actions: Sherman, D. K., & Cohen, G. L. (2006). The psychology of self-defense: Self-affirmation theory. *Advances in Experimental Social Psychology, 38,* 183-242.

Top advertising jingle: Burger Business. McDonald's Abandons 'You Deserve a Break' Rights. Nov. 11, 2014. Retrieved from <http://burger-business.com/mcdonalds-abandons-you-deserve-a-break-rights/>

Stop seeking an escape through food: Heatherton, T. F., & Baumeister, R. F. (1991). Binge eating as escape from self-awareness. *Psychological Bulletin*, *110*(1), 86.

CHAPTER 3. OUR OBESOGENIC ENVIRONMENT
A more accurate conceptualization of the obesity epidemic:
(1) Cohen, D. A. (2008). Obesity and the built environment: Changes in environmental cues cause energy imbalances. *International Journal of Obesity*, *32*, S137-S142.
(2) Cohen, D. (2013). *A big fat crisis: The hidden forces behind the obesity epidemic and how we can end it*. Nation Books.

Our modern obesogenic environment:
(1) Morris, M. J., Beilharz, J. E., Maniam, J., Reichelt, A. C., & Westbrook, R. F. (2014). Why is obesity such a problem in the 21st century? The intersection of palatable food, cues and reward pathways, stress, and cognition. *Neuroscience & Biobehavioral Reviews*, pii: S0149-7634(14)00333-9.
(2) Brownell, K. D., & Warner, K. E. (2009). The perils of ignoring history: Big Tobacco played dirty and millions died. How similar is Big Food? *Milbank Quarterly*, *87*(1), 259-294.
(3) Swinburn, B. A., Sacks, G., Hall, K. D., McPherson, K., Finegood, D. T., Moodie, M. L., & Gortmaker, S. L. (2011). The global obesity pandemic: Shaped by global drivers and local environments. *The Lancet*, *378*(9793), 804-814.

It is truly a toxic environment: Harvard School of Public Health. Toxic food environment: How our surroundings influence what we eat. Obesity Prevention Source. Retrieved from <http://www.hsph.harvard.edu/obesity-prevention-source/obesity-causes/food-environment-and-obesity/>

Between 1970 and 2000 our average calorie consumption increased: U.S. Department of Agriculture. (2003). Profiling food consumption in America. *Agriculture Fact Book 2001-2002*, Chapter 2, p. 14.

Increasingly available, cheap, obesogenic foods:
(1) *Quote from*: Swinburn, B. A., Sacks, G., Hall, K. D., McPherson, K., Finegood, D. T., Moodie, M. L., & Gortmaker, S. L. (2011). The global obesity pandemic: Shaped by global drivers and local environments. *The Lancet, 378*(9793), 804-814.
(2) Chandon, P., & Wansink, B. (2012). Does food marketing need to make us fat? A review and solutions. *Nutrition Reviews, 70*(10), 571-593.
(3) *Fat and sugar are cheap*: French, S. A. (2003). Pricing effects on food choices. *The Journal of Nutrition, 133*(3), 841S-843S.
(4) *Hyperpalatable diets are cheap*: Rehm, C. D., Monsivais, P., & Drewnowski, A. (2015). Relation between diet cost and Healthy Eating Index 2010 scores among adults in the United States 2007–2010. *Preventive Medicine, 73*, 70-75.

Ultra-processed foods & beverages make up nearly 60% of the calories and 90% of the sugar we consume: On average, *less than one-third of our calories come from unprocessed foods*: Steele, E. M., Baraldi, L. G., da Costa Louzada, M. L., Moubarac, J. C., Mozaffarian, D., & Monteiro, C. A. (2016). Ultra-processed foods and added sugars in the US diet: Evidence from a nationally representative cross-sectional study. *BMJ Open, 6*(3), e009892.

Sources of empty calories and sugar in the U.S. diet:
(1) Reedy, J., & Krebs-Smith, S. M. (2010). Dietary sources of energy, solid fats, and added sugars among children and adolescents in the United States. *Journal of the American Dietetic Association, 110*(10), 1477-1484.
(2) *One-third of daily calories come from snack foods:* Bliss, R.M. (2012). Snacking associated with increased calories, decreased nutrients. U.S. Department of Agriculture, Agricultural Research Service, March 12, 2012.
(3) *Desserts, snacks and beverages contribute 83% of added sugar:* O'Neil, C. E., Keast, D. R., Fulgoni, V. L., & Nicklas, T. A. (2012). Food sources of energy and nutrients among adults in the US: NHANES 2003–2006. *Nutrients, 4*(12), 2097-2120.
(4) *The largest sources of sugar are beverages, grain desserts, fruit drinks, candy, and dairy desserts:* Drewnowski, A., & Rehm, C. D. (2014). Consumption of

added sugars among US children and adults by food purchase location and food source. *The American Journal of Clinical Nutrition*, *100*(3), 901-907.

Sugar-sweetened beverages and the obesity epidemic:
(1) Hu, F. B. (2013). Resolved: There is sufficient scientific evidence that decreasing sugar-sweetened beverage consumption will reduce the prevalence of obesity and obesity-related diseases. *Obesity Reviews*, *14*(8), 606-619.
(2) *Consumption of sugar-sweetened beverages has increased fivefold since 1950. Approximately 75% of all foods and beverages now contain added sugar in various forms:* Bray, G. A., and Popkin, B. M. (2014). Dietary sugar and body weight: Have we reached a crisis in the epidemic of obesity and diabetes? Health be damned! Pour on the sugar. *Diabetes Care*, *37*(4), 950-956.
(3) *Sugar-sweetened sodas may contribute to metabolic disease:* Leung, C. W., Laraia, B. A., Needham, B. L., Rehkopf, D. H., Adler, N. E., Lin, J., ... & Epel, E. S. (2014). Soda and cell aging: Associations between sugar-sweetened beverage consumption and leukocyte telomere length in healthy adults from the National Health and Nutrition Examination Surveys. *American Journal of Public Health*, *104*(12), 2425-2431.

We do not eat enough fruits and vegetables, whole grains and low-fat milk products: Krebs-Smith, S. M., Reedy, J., & Bosire, C. (2010). Healthfulness of the US food supply: Little improvement despite decades of dietary guidance. *American Journal of Preventive Medicine*, *38*(5), 472-477.

A lack of physical activity is part of the obesogenic equation:
(1) Blundell, J. E., & King, N. A. (1999). Physical activity and regulation of food intake: Current evidence. *Medicine and Science in Sports and Exercise*, *31*, S573-S583.
(2) DeLany, J. P., Kelley, D. E., Hames, K. C., Jakicic, J. M., & Goodpaster, B. H. (2014). Effect of physical activity on weight loss, energy expenditure, and energy intake during diet induced weight loss. *Obesity*, *22*(2), 363-370.

Our environments are largely sedentary: *Occupation-related energy expenditure has decreased by more than 100 calories per day*: Church, T. S., Thomas, D. M., Tudor-Locke, C., Katzmarzyk, P. T., Earnest, C. P., Rodarte, R. Q., ... & Bouchard, C. (2011). Trends over 5 decades in US occupation-related physical activity and their associations with obesity. *PLoS One*, *6*(5), e19657.

Sedentary behaviors promote weight gain:
(1) *Nurse's health study*: Hu, F. B., Li, T. Y., Colditz, G. A., Willett, W. C., & Manson, J. E. (2003). Television watching and other sedentary behaviors in relation to risk of obesity and type 2 diabetes mellitus in women. *JAMA*, *289*(14), 1785-1791.
(2) *Television watching, alcohol intake, and sleep deprivation encourage excessive eating*: Chapman, C. D., Benedict, C., Brooks, S. J., & Schiöth, H. B. (2012). Lifestyle determinants of the drive to eat: A meta-analysis. *The American Journal of Clinical Nutrition*, *96*(3), 492-497.
(3) *Prolonged TV viewing is associated with an increased risk of type 2 diabetes, cardiovascular disease, and all-cause mortality*: Grøntved, A., & Hu, F. B. (2011). Television viewing and risk of type 2 diabetes, cardiovascular disease, and all-cause mortality: A meta-analysis. *JAMA*, *305*(23), 2448-2455.
(4) *Television advertising is associated with obesity in children*: Zimmerman, F. J., & Bell, J. F. (2010). Associations of television content type and obesity in children. *American Journal of Public Health*, *100*(2), 334.
(5) *Screen time is associated with increased consumption of foods high in fat, sugar or salt*: Börnhorst, C., Wijnhoven, T. M., Kunešová, M., Yngve, A., Rito, A. I., Lissner, L., ... & Breda, J. (2015). WHO European Childhood Obesity Surveillance Initiative: Associations between sleep duration, screen time and food consumption frequencies. *BMC Public Health*, *15*(1), 442.

We eat more hyperpalatable food when we are sedentary: Chaput, J. P., Klingenberg, L., Astrup, A., & Sjödin, A. M. (2011). Modern sedentary activities promote overconsumption of food in our current obesogenic environment. *Obesity Reviews*, *12*(5), e12-e20.

A lack of sleep is strongly associated with hunger, overeating, weight gain:
(1) Van Cauter, E., & Knutson, K. L. (2008). Sleep and the epidemic of obesity in children and adults. *European Journal of Endocrinology*, *159*(suppl 1), S59-S66.
(2) Penev, P. D. (2012). Update on energy homeostasis and insufficient sleep. *The Journal of Clinical Endocrinology & Metabolism*, *97*(6), 1792-1801.
(3) Chaput, J. P. (2014). Sleep patterns, diet quality and energy balance. *Physiology & Behavior*, *134*, 86-91.
(4) *Shorter sleep duration is associated with increased weight*: Watson, N. F., Harden, K. P., Buchwald, D., Vitiello, M. V., Pack, A. I., Weigle, D. S., & Goldberg, J. (2012). Sleep duration and body mass index in twins: A gene-environment interaction. *Sleep*, *35*(5), 597.
(5) *In the Quebec Family Study, the best predictor of future obesity was short sleep duration*: Chaput, J. P., Leblanc, C., Pérusse, L., Després, J. P., Bouchard, C., & Tremblay, A. (2009). Risk factors for adult overweight and obesity in the Quebec Family Study: Have we been barking up the wrong tree? *Obesity*, *17*(10), 1964-1970.

Americans are not getting enough sleep:
(1) National Sleep Foundation. Lack of sleep is affecting Americans, finds the National Sleep Foundation. Dec. 2014. Retrieved from <https://sleepfoundation.org/media-center/press-release/lack-sleep-affecting-americans-finds-the-national-sleep-foundation>
(2) Basner, M., Fomberstein, K. M., Razavi, F. M., Banks, S., William, J. H., Rosa, R. R., & Dinges, D. F. (2007). American time use survey: Sleep time and its relationship to waking activities. *Sleep*, *30*(9), 1085.
(3) *35% of adults reported less than 7 hours of sleep per day:* Centers for Disease Control and Prevention. (2015). Insufficient sleep is a public health epidemic. Retrieved from <http://www.cdc.gov/features/dssleep/>
(4) American Psychological Association. More sleep would make most Americans happier, healthier and safer. Feb. 2014. Retrieved from <http://www.apa.org/action/resources/research-in-action/sleep-deprivation.aspx>

People are more inclined to snack on junk foods when they are sleep-deprived:
(1) St-Onge, M. P., McReynolds, A., Trivedi, Z. B., Roberts, A. L., Sy, M., & Hirsch, J. (2012). Sleep restriction leads to increased activation of brain regions sensitive to food stimuli. *The American Journal of Clinical Nutrition*, *95*(4), 818-824.
(2) Nedeltcheva, A. V., Kilkus, J. M., Imperial, J., Kasza, K., Schoeller, D. A., & Penev, P. D. (2009). Sleep curtailment is accompanied by increased intake of calories from snacks. *The American Journal of Clinical Nutrition*, *89*(1), 126-133.
(3) Weiss, A., Xu, F., Storfer-Isser, A., Thomas, A., Ievers-Landis, C. E., & Redline, S. (2010). The association of sleep duration with adolescents' fat and carbohydrate consumption. *Sleep*, *33*(9), 1201.

One reason cited for snacking is "to gain energy": Verhoeven, A. A., Adriaanse, M. A., de Vet, E., Fennis, B. M., & de Ridder, D. T. (2015). It's my party and I eat if I want to: Reasons for unhealthy snacking. *Appetite*, *84*, 20-27.

A lack of sleep plays havoc with ghrelin, leptin, and appetite:
(1) Greer, S. M., Goldstein, A. N., & Walker, M. P. (2013). The impact of sleep deprivation on food desire in the human brain. *Nature Communications*, *4*, 2259.
(2) Galli, G., Piaggi, P., Mattingly, M. S., de Jonge, L., Courville, A. B., Pinchera, A., ... & Cizza, G. (2013). Inverse relationship of food and alcohol intake to sleep measures in obesity. *Nutrition & Diabetes*, *3*(1), e58.
(3) Taheri, S., Lin, L., Austin, D., Young, T., & Mignot, E. (2004). Short sleep duration is associated with reduced leptin, elevated ghrelin, and increased body mass index. *PLoS Medicine*, *1*(3), e62.
(4) Killgore, W. D., Schwab, Z. J., Weber, M., Kipman, M., DelDonno, S. R., Weiner, M. R., & Rauch, S. L. (2013). Daytime sleepiness affects prefrontal regulation of food intake. *Neuroimage*, *71*, 216-223.

(5) Chaput, J. P., Despres, J. P., Bouchard, C., & Tremblay, A. (2012). Longer sleep duration associates with lower adiposity gain in adult short sleepers. *International Journal of Obesity*, 36(5), 752-756.
(6) Penev, P. D. (2012). Update on energy homeostasis and insufficient sleep. *The Journal of Clinical Endocrinology & Metabolism*, 97(6), 1792-1801.

More than two-thirds of Americans are overweight or obese: Ogden, C.L., Carroll, M.D., Kit, B.K., & Flegal, K.M. Prevalence of obesity in the United States, 2009–2010. *Centers for Disease Control and Prevention*. Retrieved from <http://www.cdc.gov/nchs/fastats/obesity-overweight.htm>

The rising tide of obesity, a tsunami:
(1) *The environmental tsunami of cues prompts people to overconsume:* Cohen, D. A. (2008). Obesity and the built environment: Changes in environmental cues cause energy imbalances. *International Journal of Obesity*, 32, S137-S142.
(2) Finucane, M. M., Stevens, G. A., Cowan, M. J., Danaei, G., Lin, J. K., Paciorek, C. J., ... & Global Burden of Metabolic Risk Factors of Chronic Diseases Collaborating Group (Body Mass Index.) (2011). National, regional, and global trends in body-mass index since 1980: Systematic analysis of health examination surveys and epidemiological studies with 960 country-years and 9.1 million participants. *The Lancet*, 377(9765), 557-567.
(3) Olshansky, S. J., Passaro, D. J., Hershow, R. C., Layden, J., Carnes, B. A., Brody, J., ... & Ludwig, D. S. (2005). A potential decline in life expectancy in the United States in the 21st century. *New England Journal of Medicine*, 352(11), 1138-1145.
(4) Children's Hospital Boston. (2005). Explosion of child obesity predicted to shorten U.S. life expectancy. *ScienceDaily*, March 2005. Retrieved from <www.sciencedaily.com/releases/2005/03/050325144425.htm>

Obesity increases the risk for diabetes, heart disease and other diseases:
(1)Wild, S. H., & Byrne, C. D. (2006). ABC of obesity: Risk factors for diabetes and coronary heart disease. *BMJ: British Medical Journal*, *333*(7576), 1009.
(2) Johnson, R. K., Appel, L. J., Brands, M., Howard, B. V., Lefevre, M., Lustig, R. H., ... & Wylie-Rosett, J. (2009). Dietary sugars intake and cardiovascular health: A scientific statement from the American Heart Association. *Circulation*, *120*(11), 1011-1020.
(3) DiNicolantonio, J. J., & Lucan, S. C. (2014). The wrong white crystals: Not salt but sugar as aetiological in hypertension and cardiometabolic disease. *Open Heart*, *1*(1), e000167.
(4) National Heart, Lung and Blood Institute (NIH). What Are the Health Risks of Overweight and Obesity? Updated July 13, 2012. Retrieved from <https://www.nhlbi.nih.gov/health/health-topics/topics/obe/risks>

Obesity is spreading around the globe: *The number of obese people has risen from 105 million in 1975 to 641 million in 2014. By 2025, approximately 20% of adults worldwide will be obese*: Ezzati, M., & NCD Risk Factor Collaboration. (2016). Trends in adult body-mass index in 200 countries from 1975 to 2014: A pooled analysis of 1698 population-based measurement studies with 19.2 million participants. *The Lancet*, *387*(10026), 1377–96.

McKinsey Report: Dobbs, R., Sawers, C., Thompson, F., Manyika, J., Woetzel, J., Child, P., McKenna, S., & Spatharou, A. (2014). How the world could better fight obesity. McKinsey & Company, Nov 2014. Retrieved from <http://www.mckinsey.com/insights/economic_studies/how_the_world_could_better_fight_obesity>

Fast foods loaded with calories are often eaten at lunch or dinner:
(1)Dugan, A. (2013). Fast food still major part of U.S. diet: Gallup's annual consumption poll, conducted July 10-14, 2013. Retrieved from <http://www.gallup.com/poll/163868/fast-food-major-part-diet.aspx>

(2) *Americans consume one third of their daily calories from foods prepared outside the home, where portion sizes have expanded greatly*: Economic Research Service. (2010). Food marketing system in the U.S.: Food service. Washington DC: U.S. Department of Agriculture. Retrieved from <www.ers.usda.gov/Briefing/FoodMarketingSystem/foodservice.htm>

(3) *Fast-food consumption contributes to increased calorie intake:* Rosenheck, R. (2008). Fast food consumption and increased caloric intake: A systematic review of a trajectory towards weight gain and obesity risk. *Obesity Reviews, 9*(6), 535-547.

Portion sizes have increased over time:
(1) Nestle, M. (2003). Increasing portion sizes in American diets: More calories, more obesity. *Journal of the American Dietetic Association, 103*(1), 39-40.

(2) Young, L. R., & Nestle, M. (2012). Reducing portion sizes to prevent obesity: A call to action. *American Journal of Preventive Medicine, 43*(5), 565-568.

The average meal out contains 1000-1500 calories:
(1) *The average meal contains 1,327 calories:* Urban, L. E., Lichtenstein, A. H., Gary, C. E., Fierstein, J. L., Equi, A., Kussmaul, C., ... & Roberts, S. B. (2013). The energy content of restaurant foods without stated calorie information. *JAMA Internal Medicine, 173*(14), 1292-1299.

(2) *Per meal, teens ate 1,038 calories at McDonald's and 955 calories at Subway*: Lesser, L. I., Kayekjian, K. C., Velasquez, P., Tseng, C. H., Brook, R. H., & Cohen, D. A. (2013). Adolescent purchasing behavior at McDonald's and Subway. *Journal of Adolescent Health, 53*(4), 441-445.

(3) *Adult meals at full-service restaurant chains contained approximately 1,495 kcal before the beverage*: Auchincloss, A. H., Leonberg, B. L., Glanz, K., Bellitz, S., Ricchezza, A., & Jervis, A. (2014). Nutritional value of meals at full-service restaurant chains. *Journal of Nutrition Education and Behavior, 46*(1), 75-81.

The more often people eat fast food, the greater their chances of gaining weight: Pereira, M. A., Kartashov, A. I., Ebbeling, C. B., Van Horn, L., Slattery, M. L., Jacobs, D. R., & Ludwig, D. S. (2005). Fast-food habits, weight gain, and insulin resistance (the CARDIA study): 15-year prospective analysis. *The Lancet, 365*(9453), 36-42.

The amount of food we eat increases *as the effort to obtain it* decreases: (1) Wansink, B. (2004). Environmental factors that increase the food intake and consumption volume of unknowing consumers. *Annu. Rev. Nutr., 24,* 455-479. (2) *The foods that have shown the greatest increase in sales are those that require the least effort to obtain and to eat*: Nielsen, S. J., Siega-Riz, A. M., & Popkin, B. M. (2002). Trends in energy intake in US between 1977 and 1996: Similar shifts seen across age groups. *Obesity Research, 10*(5), 370-378.

People given larger portions eat more food:
(1) *Larger portions lead to substantial increases in energy intake*: Rolls, B. J. (2014). What is the role of portion control in weight management? *International Journal of Obesity, 38,* S1-S8.
(2) *The effect of portion size on energy intake is particularly pronounced with energy-dense foods*: Livingstone, M. B. E., & Pourshahidi, L. K. (2014). Portion size and obesity. *Advances in Nutrition: An International Review Journal, 5*(6), 829-834.
(3)*Dinnerware size serves as a consumption norm*: Wansink, B., & Van Ittersum, K. (2007). Portion size me: Downsizing our consumption norms. *Journal of the American Dietetic Association, 107*(7), 1103-1106.
(4) *When given a large bowl, diners served themselves more pasta*: Van Kleef, E., Shimizu, M., & Wansink, B. (2012). Serving bowl selection biases the amount of food served. *Journal of Nutrition Education and Behavior, 44*(1), 66-70.
(5) *Individuals presented with large portions generally do not respond to increased levels of fullness*: Ello-Martin, J. A., Ledikwe, J. H., & Rolls, B. J. (2005). The influence of food portion size and energy density on energy intake:

Implications for weight management. *The American Journal of Clinical Nutrition*, *82*(1), 236S-241S.

People who were served 50% more pasta ate 43% more: Diliberti, N., Bordi, P. L., Conklin, M. T., Roe, L. S., & Rolls, B. J. (2004). Increased portion size leads to increased energy intake in a restaurant meal. *Obesity Research*, *12*(3),562-8.

Studies published by Dr. Brian Wansink: Wansink, Brian, Ph.D. (2006). *Mindless eating: Why we eat more than we think*. New York: Bantam Books. Website: http://mindlesseating.org/

People consume more than 90% of the food on their plate: Wansink, B., & Johnson, K. A. (2014). The clean plate club: About 92% of self-served food is eaten. *International Journal of Obesity*, 39, 371–374.

People given large portions did not believe they had eaten more:
(1) Wansink, B., Just, D., & Payne, C. R. (2009). Mindless eating and healthy heuristics for the irrational. *American Economic Review*, *99*, 165.
(2) *We don't want to believe that our behavior is automatic*: Bargh, J. A., & Chartrand, T. L. (1999). The unbearable automaticity of being. *American Psychologist*, *54*(7), 462.

Smaller portions can be equally satisfying: Van Kleef, E., Shimizu, M., & Wansink, B. (2013). Just a bite: Considerably smaller snack portions satisfy delayed hunger and craving. *Food Quality and Preference*, *27*(1), 96-100.

Potato chip consumption has gone up:
(1) Sterk, R. Potato chip consumption up despite focus on healthy foods. *Food Business News*, April 29, 2008, p. 23.
(2) *Potatoes are typically consumed in ways that add fat and calories*: Guthrie, J., & Lin, B.-H. (2014). Healthy vegetables undermined by the company

they keep. U.S. Department of Agriculture, May 5, 2014. Retrieved from <http://www.ers.usda.gov/amber-waves/2014-may/healthy-vegetables-undermined-by-the-company-they-keep.aspx#.VsEXnObHmzU>

Potato chip consumption increases as the package size increases: Rolls, B. J., Roe, L. S., Kral, T. V., Meengs, J. S., & Wall, D. E. (2004). Increasing the portion size of a packaged snack increases energy intake in men and women. *Appetite*, *42*(1), 63-69.

The power of the potato chip:
(1) Hoch, T., Kreitz, S., Gaffling, S., Pischetsrieder, M., & Hess, A. (2013). Manganese-enhanced magnetic resonance imaging for mapping of whole brain activity patterns associated with the intake of snack food in ad libitum fed rats. *PloS One*, *8*(2), e55354.
(2) Hoch, T., Pischetsrieder, M., & Hess, A. (2014). Snack food intake in ad libitum fed rats is triggered by the combination of fat and carbohydrates. *Frontiers in Psychology*, *5*, 250.
(3) Hoch, T., Kreitz, S., Gaffling, S., Pischetsrieder, M., & Hess, A. (2015). Fat/carbohydrate ratio but not energy density determines snack food intake and activates brain reward areas. *Scientific Reports*, *5*, 10041.

Hedonic hyperphagia (eating for pleasure rather than for need): Monteleone, P., Piscitelli, F., Scognamiglio, P., Monteleone, A. M., Canestrelli, B., Di Marzo, V., & Maj, M. (2012). Hedonic eating is associated with increased peripheral levels of ghrelin and the endocannabinoid 2-arachidonoyl-glycerol in healthy humans: A pilot study. *The Journal of Clinical Endocrinology & Metabolism*, *97*(6), E917-E924.

Foods that are high in fat, sugar, and salt stimulate the appetite:
(1) *Sugar and fat have synergistic effects*: Drenowski, A., & Almiron-Roig, E. Human perceptions and preferences for fat-rich foods. *Fat Detection: Taste, Texture, and Post Ingestive Effects*, edited by J.P. Montmayeur and J. le Coutre. Boca Raton (FL): CRC Press, 2010.

(2) Hariri, N., Gougeon, R., and Thibault, L. (2010). A highly saturated fat-rich diet is more obesogenic than diets with lower saturated fat content. *Nutrition Research*, *30*(9), 632-643.

Dr. Ashley Gearhardt: Gearhardt, A. N., Grilo, C. M., DiLeone, R. J., Brownell, K. D., & Potenza, M. N. (2011). Can food be addictive? Public health and policy implications. *Addiction*, *106*(7), 1208-1212.

Maltodextrin: *Maltodextrin causes an insulin response similar to that of glucose*: Smeets, P. A., de Graaf, C., Stafleu, A., van Osch, M. J., & van der Grond, J. (2005). Functional magnetic resonance imaging of human hypothalamic responses to sweet taste and calories. *The American Journal of Clinical Nutrition*, *82*(5), 1011-1016.

The glycemic index of foods is associated with reward-driven eating:
(1) Brand-Miller, J., Atkinson, F., & Rowan, A. (2013). Effect of added carbohydrates on glycemic and insulin responses to children's milk products. *Nutrients*, *5*(1), 23-31.
(2) Ludwig DS. The glycemic index: Physiological mechanisms relating to obesity, diabetes, and cardiovascular disease. *JAMA 2002;287:2414–23.*
(3) Lennerz, B. S., Alsop, D. C., Holsen, L. M., Stern, E., Rojas, R., Ebbeling, C. B., ... & Ludwig, D. S. (2013). Effects of dietary glycemic index on brain regions related to reward and craving in men. *The American Journal of Clinical Nutrition*, *98*(3), 641-647.
(4) *Glycemic index should not be used in isolation; the energy density and macronutrient profile should also be considered*: Atkinson, F. S., Foster-Powell, K., & Brand-Miller, J. C. (2008). International tables of glycemic index and glycemic load values: 2008. *Diabetes Care*, *31*(12), 2281-2283.

Link between highly processed foods and overeating/addiction:
(1) Schulte, E. M., Avena, N. M., & Gearhardt, A. N. (2015). Which foods may be addictive? The roles of processing, fat content, and glycemic load. *PloS One*, *10*(2), e0117959.

(2) Davis, C. (2014). Evolutionary and neuropsychological perspectives on addictive behaviors and addictive substances: Relevance to the 'food addiction' construct. *Substance Abuse and Rehabilitation, 5*, 129.

(3) *White bread increases the risk of weight gain:* de la Fuente-Arrillaga, C., Martinez-Gonzalez, M. A., Zazpe-Garcia, I., Vazquez-Ruiz, Z., Benito-Corchon, S., & Bes-Rastrollo, M. (2014). Glycemic load, glycemic index, bread and incidence of overweight/obesity in a Mediterranean cohort: The SUN project. *BMC Public Health, 14*(1), 1091.

MSG is associated with weight gain: He, K., Du, S., Xun, P., Sharma, S., Wang, H., Zhai, F., & Popkin, B. (2011). Consumption of monosodium glutamate in relation to incidence of overweight in Chinese adults: China Health and Nutrition Survey (CHNS). *The American Journal of Clinical Nutrition, 93*(6), 1328-1336.

Eating is often an automatic reaction to the environment:
(1) *80% of eating episodes have nothing to do with hunger:* Tuomisto, T., Tuomisto, M. T., Hetherington, M., & Lappalainen, R. (1998). Reasons for initiation and cessation of eating in obese men and women and the affective consequences of eating in everyday situations. *Appetite, 30*(2), 211-222.

(2) de Castro, J. M., King, G. A., Duarte-Gardea, M., Gonzalez-Ayala, S., & Kooshian, C. H. (2012). Overweight and obese humans overeat away from home. *Appetite, 59*(2), 204-211.

(3) Seguin, R. A., Aggarwal, A., Vermeylen, F., & Drewnowski, A. (2016). Consumption frequency of foods away from home linked with higher body mass index and lower fruit and vegetable intake among adults: A cross-sectional study. *Journal of Environmental and Public Health, 2016* (2016), Article ID 3074241.

Sugar is the main culprit, and when sugar is combined with fat the effects are magnified:
(1) Ahmed, S. H. Is sugar as addictive as cocaine? *Food and Addiction: A Comprehensive Handbook*. Oxford University Press, 2012.

(2) *A particular hedonic synergy is obtained by combining sugar and fat*: Drewnowski, A., & Almiron-Roig, E. Human perceptions and preferences for fat-rich foods. *Fat Detection: Taste, Texture, and Post Ingestive Effects*, edited by J.P. Montmayeur and J. le Coutre. Boca Raton (FL): CRC Press, 2010.

(3) Hariri, N., Gougeon, R., & Thibault, L. (2010). A highly saturated fat-rich diet is more obesogenic than diets with lower saturated fat content. *Nutrition Research, 30*(9), 632-643.

(4) *Fats and sugars in combination predicted increases in BMI*: Lindberg, M. A., Dementieva, Y., & Cavender, J. (2011). Why has the BMI gone up so drastically in the last 35 years? *Journal of Addiction Medicine, 5*(4), 272-278.

(5) *Sucrose is the dominant reinforcing component*: Naleid, A. M., Grimm, J. W., Kessler, D. A., Sipols, A. J., Aliakbari, S., Bennett, J. L., ... & Figlewicz, D. P. (2008). Deconstructing the vanilla milkshake: The dominant effect of sucrose on self-administration of nutrient–flavor mixtures. *Appetite, 50*(1), 128-138.

The consumption of added sugars has increased:

(1) *Per capita consumption of caloric sweeteners increased by 43 pounds per year between 1950-59 and 2000:* U.S. Department of Agriculture. (2003). Profiling food consumption in America. *Agriculture Fact Book 2001-2002*, March 2003.

(2) Wells, H.F., & Buzby, J.C. Dietary assessment of major trends in U.S. food consumption, 1970-2005. United States Department of Agriculture, Economic Research Service. *Economic Information Bulletin, 33*, March 2008.

(3) *The top 20% of adult consumers consume 721 calories from added sugar per day*: The Obesity Society. (2014). U.S. adult consumption of added sugars increased by more than 30% over three decades. Press Release, Nov 4, 2014. Retrieved from <http://www.prnewswire.com/news-releases/us-adult-consumption-of-added-sugars-increased-by-more-than-30-over-three-decades-281475601.html>

(4) Center for Science in the Public Interest. Sugar: Too much of a sweet thing: Infographic. Retrieved from <http://cspinet.org/new/pdf/combined_infographic.pdf>.

Recommendation to limit added sugars: World Health Organization. (2015). WHO calls on countries to reduce sugars intake among adults and children. Press release, March 4, 2015. Retrieved from <http://www.who.int/mediacentre/news/releases/2015/sugar-guideline/en/>

Nearly 60% of the population exceeds the recommended limits for added sugar: Baraldi, L. G., da Costa Louzada, M. L., Moubarac, J. C., Mozaffarian, D., & Monteiro, C. A. (2016). Ultra-processed foods and added sugars in the US diet: Evidence from a nationally representative cross-sectional study. *BMJ Open, 6*(3), e009892.

Sugar consumption is linked to diabetes and cardiovascular disease:
(1) Basu, S., Yoffe, P., Hills, N., & Lustig, R. H. (2013). The relationship of sugar to population-level diabetes prevalence: an econometric analysis of repeated cross-sectional data. *PLoS One, 8*(2), e57873.
(2) de Koning L., Malik, V. S., Rimm, E. B., Willett, W. C., & Hu, F. B. (2011). Sugar-sweetened and artificially sweetened beverage consumption and risk of type 2 diabetes in men. *The American Journal of Clinical Nutrition, 93*(6), 1321-1327.
(3) Yang Q., Zhang, Z., Gregg, E. W., Flanders, W. D., Merritt, R., & Hu, F. B. (2014). Added sugar intake and cardiovascular diseases mortality among US adults. *JAMA Internal Medicine, 174*(4), 516-524.

Foods that are cited as being craved are those with high amounts of sugar and fat:
Gilhooly, C. H., Das, S. K., Golden, J. K., McCrory, M. A., Dallal, G. E., Saltzman, E., ... & Roberts, S. B. (2007). Food cravings and energy regulation: The characteristics of craved foods and their relationship with eating behaviors and weight change during 6 months of dietary energy restriction. *International Journal of Obesity, 31*(12), 1849-1858.

CHAPTER 4. WHY WE OVEREAT
Effective weight-loss involves delaying, changing, and shifting automatic behaviors as well as planning and implementing new eating and

activity choices: Inzlicht, M., Legault, L., & Teper, R. (2014). Exploring the mechanisms of self-control improvement. *Current Directions in Psychological Science*, *23*(4), 302-307.

Homeostatic and non-homeostatic systems control food intake: Lutter, M., & Nestler, E. J. (2009). Homeostatic and hedonic signals interact in the regulation of food intake. *The Journal of Nutrition*, *139*(3), 629-632.

Reward-driven eating strongly contributes to weight gain and obesity:
(1) Berridge, K. C., Ho, C. Y., Richard, J. M., & DiFeliceantonio, A. G. (2010). The tempted brain eats: Pleasure and desire circuits in obesity and eating disorders. Brain research, 1350, 43-64.
(2) Kenny, P. J. (2011). Reward mechanisms in obesity: New insights and future directions. *Neuron*, *69*(4), 664-679.
(3) Murray, S., Tulloch, A., Gold, M. S., & Avena, N. M. (2014). Hormonal and neural mechanisms of food reward, eating behaviour and obesity. *Nature Reviews Endocrinology*, *10*(9), 540.

When pleasurable eating occurs there is a release of dopamine in the reward center:
(1) Castro, D. C., & Berridge, K. C. (2014). Advances in the neurobiological bases for food 'liking' versus 'wanting'. *Physiology & Behavior*, *136*, 22-30.
(2) Baik, J. H. (2013). Dopamine signaling in reward-related behaviors. *Front Neural Circuits*, 7, 152.
(3) Saunders, B. T., Richard, J. M., & Janak, P. H. (2015). Contemporary approaches to neural circuit manipulation and mapping: focus on reward and addiction. *Phil. Trans. R. Soc. B*, *370*(1677), 20140210.

The reward system can motivate us to eat even when we are not hungry:
(1) Berthoud, H. R. (2012). The neurobiology of food intake in an obesogenic environment. *Proceedings of the Nutrition Society*, *71*(04), 478-487.

(2) *Environmental cues that acquire motivational properties can subsequently override satiety:* Petrovich, G. D., & Gallagher, M. (2007). Control of food consumption by learned cues: A forebrain–hypothalamic network. *Physiology & Behavior, 91*(4), 397-403.

(3) *There is nothing "wrong" with the system, it is merely overwhelmed by its environment:* Hall, K. D., Hammond, R. A., & Rahmandad, H. (2014). Dynamic interplay among homeostatic, hedonic, and cognitive feedback circuits regulating body weight. *American Journal of Public Health, 104*(7), 1169-1175.

(4) *Signaling mechanisms that initiate a meal are generally nonhomeostatic:* Alonso-Alonso, M., Woods, S. C., Pelchat, M., Grigson, P. S., Stice, E., Farooqi, S., ... & Beauchamp, G. K. (2015). Food reward system: Current perspectives and future research needs. *Nutrition Reviews, 73*(5), 296-307.

Functional MRI, brain response to images of hyperpalatable food:
(1) Perello, M., Chuang, J. C., Scott, M. M., & Lutter, M. (2010). Translational neuroscience approaches to hyperphagia. *The Journal of Neuroscience, 30*(35), 11549-11554.

(2) Gearhardt, A. N., Yokum, S., Orr, P. T., Stice, E., Corbin, W. R., & Brownell, K. D. (2011). Neural correlates of food addiction. *Archives of General Psychiatry, 68*(8), 808-816.

(3) Pelchat, M. L., Johnson, A., Chan, R., Valdez, J., & Ragland, J. D. (2004). Images of desire: Food-craving activation during fMRI. *Neuroimage, 23*(4), 1486-1493.

The more desirable something is, the more significant the changes:
(1) *An interview with Harvard University's Dr. Uma Karmarkar:* Nobel, C. What neuroscience tells us about consumer desire. *Harvard Business School Working Knowledge*, March 26, 2012. Copyright 2012 President and Fellows of Harvard College. Retrieved from <http://hbswk.hbs.edu/item/6950.html>

(2) *Activation of the insula and the nucleus accumbens could predict the decision to buy a wide range of consumer products:* Knutson, B., Rick, S., Wimmer, G.

E., Prelec, D., & Loewenstein, G. (2007). Neural predictors of purchases. *Neuron, 53*(1), 147-156.

(3) *The good news: Using a neurofeedback system, participants were able to successfully down-regulate individually defined target areas*: Sokunbi, M. O., Linden, D. E., Habes, I., Johnston, S., & Ihssen, N. (2014). Real-time fMRI brain-computer interface: Development of a 'motivational feedback' subsystem for the regulation of visual cue reactivity. *Frontiers in Behavioral Neuroscience, 8,* 392.

The 'hot' system described by Metcalfe and Mischel: *The dual-process model describes temptations as hot, impulsive forces that can be counteracted by rational, "top down" processes*: Metcalfe, J., & Mischel, W. (1999). A hot/cool-system analysis of delay of gratification: Dynamics of willpower. *Psychological Review, 106*(1), 3.

It is not necessary to consume the food to activate the reward center: *Distinct circuits respond to pictures of food versus receipt of food*: D'Agostino, A. E., & Small, D. M. (2012). Neuroimaging the interaction of mind and metabolism in humans. *Molecular Metabolism, 1*(1), 10-20.

Images of hyperpalatable food can trigger overeating:
(1) Stoeckel LE, Weller, R. E., Cook, E. W., Twieg, D. B., Knowlton, R. C., & Cox, J. E. (2008). Widespread reward-system activation in obese women in response to pictures of high-calorie foods. *Neuroimage, 41*(2), 636-647.

(2) *Food cues and subsequent snack food consumption:* Lawrence, N. S., Hinton, E. C., Parkinson, J. A., & Lawrence, A. D. (2012). Nucleus accumbens response to food cues predicts subsequent snack consumption in women and increased body mass index in those with reduced self-control. *Neuroimage, 63*(1), 415-422.

(3) *Association between neural activation and BMI:* Simon, J. J., Skunde, M., Sinno, M. H., Brockmeyer, T., Herpertz, S. C., Bendszus, M., ... & Friederich, H. C. (2014). Impaired cross-talk between mesolimbic food reward processing and metabolic signaling predicts body mass index. *Frontiers in Behavioral Neuroscience, 8.*

(4) Murdaugh, D. L., Cox, J. E., Cook, E. W., & Weller, R. E. (2012). fMRI reactivity to high-calorie food pictures predicts short-and long-term outcome in a weight-loss program. *Neuroimage, 59*(3), 2709-2721.

(5) *Even a brief exposure to the sight and smell of food increases perceived hunger*: Nederkoorn, C., Smulders, F. T. Y., & Jansen, A. (2000). Cephalic phase responses, craving and food intake in normal subjects. *Appetite, 35*(1), 45-55.

We make over 200 food decisions every day:
(1) *People make more than 200 food- and beverage-related decisions each day*: Wansink, B., & Sobal, J. (2007). Mindless eating: The 200 daily food decisions we overlook. *Environment and Behavior, 39*(1), 106-123.

(2) *Study participants indicated almost 60% more desires for unhealthy foods than healthy foods:* (a) Hofmann, W., Baumeister, R. F., Förster, G., & Vohs, K. D. (2012). Everyday temptations: An experience sampling study of desire, conflict, and self-control. *Journal of Personality and Social Psychology, 102*(6), 1318. (b) Hofmann, W., Adriaanse, M., Vohs, K. D., & Baumeister, R. F. (2014). Dieting and the self-control of eating in everyday environments: An experience sampling study. *British Journal of Health Psychology, 19*(3), 523-539.

Many people succumb to the temptation to overeat:
(1) *When Americans are asked to recall the last time they overate to the point of regret, 83% had done it within the past 10 days*: Wansink, B., & Chandon, P. (2014). Slim by design: Redirecting the accidental drivers of mindless overeating. *Journal of Consumer Psychology, 24*(3), 413-431.

(2) *Easy access to unhealthy food was associated with higher consumption in adolescents*: de Vet, E., de Wit, J. B., Luszczynska, A., Stok, F. M., Gaspar, T., Pratt, M., ... & de Ridder, D. T. (2013). Access to excess: How do adolescents deal with unhealthy foods in their environment? *European Journal of Public Health, 23*(5), 752.

The combination of sugar plus fat is particularly potent:
(1) Schroeder, J.A., Honohan, J.C., Markson, R.H., Cameron, L., Bantis, K. S., & Lopez, G. C. Nucleus accumbens c-fos expression is correlated with

conditioned place preference to cocaine, morphine and high fat/sugar food consumption. *Society for Neuroscience*, November 13, 2013.

(2) Greene, D., and NBC News staff. Addicted to Oreos? You truly might be. Today Health, Oct. 15, 2013. Retrieved from <http://www.today.com/health/addicted-oreos-you-truly-might-be-8C11399682>

(3) Cruz, J. D., Coke, T., Karagiorgis, T., Sampson, C., Icaza-Cukali, D., Kest, K., ... & Bodnar, R. J. (2015). c-Fos induction in mesotelencephalic dopamine pathway projection targets and dorsal striatum following oral intake of sugars and fats in rats. *Brain Research Bulletin*, *111*, 9-19.

(4) Levine, A. S., Kotz, C. M., & Gosnell, B. A. (2003). Sugars and fats: The neurobiology of preference. *The Journal of Nutrition*, *133*(3), 831S-834S.

(5) *Opioid effects are most potent for foods that are sweet or fatty (or both):* Taha, S. A. (2010). Preference or fat? Revisiting opioid effects on food intake. *Physiology & Behavior*, *100*(5), 429-437.

Routine overeating can lead to adaptations in the reward center:

(1) *Frequent consumption of ice cream reduces reward-region responsivity in humans, paralleling the tolerance observed in drug addiction:* Burger, K. S., & Stice, E. (2012). Frequent ice cream consumption is associated with reduced striatal response to receipt of an ice cream–based milkshake. *The American Journal of Clinical Nutrition*, *95*(4), 810-817.

(2) Lopez, R. B., Hofmann, W., Wagner, D. D., Kelley, W. M., & Heatherton, T. F. (2014). Neural predictors of giving in to temptation in daily life. *Psychological Science*, 0956797614531492.

(3) Johnson, P. M., & Kenny, P. J. (2010). Dopamine D2 receptors in addiction-like reward dysfunction and compulsive eating in obese rats. *Nature Neuroscience*, *13*(5), 635-641.

(4) *The downregulation of the µ-opioid receptor system in obesity is in accordance with that observed in opiate addictions*: Karlsson, H. K., Tuominen, L., Tuulari, J. J., Hirvonen, J., Parkkola, R., Helin, S., ... & Nummenmaa, L. (2015). Obesity is associated with decreased µ-opioid but unaltered dopamine D2 receptor availability in the brain. *The Journal of Neuroscience*, *35*(9), 3959-3965.

Dr. Kelly Brownell: "Everybody knows that some food products are intensely palatable, or habit forming... Just like drugs of abuse, brain-rewarding effects or reinforcement from food products can lead to loss of control." Brownell, K., & Gold, M. (2012). Food products. Addiction. Also in the mind [Commentary]. *World Nutrition 3*(9), 392-405.

The loss of control is rooted in biology:
(1) Lenoir, M., Serre, F., Cantin, L., & Ahmed, S. H. (2007). Intense sweetness surpasses cocaine reward. *PLoS One, 2*(8):e698.

(2) *Cocaine and food cues activate similar pathways*: Tomasi, D., Wang, G. J., Wang, R., Caparelli, E. C., Logan, J., & Volkow, N. D. (2015). Overlapping patterns of brain activation to food and cocaine cues in cocaine abusers. *Human Brain Mapping, 36*(1), 120-136.

(3) *Sweet reward is more reinforcing and attractive than either cocaine or heroin*: Madsen, H. B., & Ahmed, S. H. (2015). Drug versus sweet reward: Greater attraction to and preference for sweet versus drug cues. *Addiction biology, 20*(3), 433-444.

(4) *Rats ate more Oreo cookies than chow. When rats were placed in an environment they associated with Oreo cookies, they also ate more of a less-palatable food. Just as drug-associated context cues can reinstate drug-addiction relapse, palatable food-paired cues may trigger overeating, weight regain and obesity*: Boggiano, M. M., Dorsey, J. R., Thomas, J. M., & Murdaugh, D. L. (2009). The Pavlovian power of palatable food: Lessons for weight-loss adherence from a new rodent model of cue-induced overeating. *International Journal of Obesity, 33*(6), 693-701.

(5) *It is the brain's desire for calories that dominates our desire for sugars*: Tellez, L. A., Han, W., Zhang, X., Ferreira, T. L., Perez, I. O., Shammah-Lagnado, S. J., ... & de Araujo, I. E. (2016). Separate circuitries encode the hedonic and nutritional values of sugar. *Nature Neuroscience, 19*(3), 465-470.

Compulsive overeaters and drug users experience cravings:
(1) *Craving, a core feature of drug addiction*: Koob, G. F., & Volkow, N. D. (2010). Neurocircuitry of addiction. *Neuropsychopharmacology, 35*(1), 217-238.

(2) Blum, K., Liu, Y., Shriner, R., & S Gold, M. (2011). Reward circuitry dopaminergic activation regulates food and drug craving behavior. *Current Pharmaceutical Design*, *17*(12), 1158-1167.

Neuromarketing involves studying subconscious brain activity:
(1) *Marketing to consumers sometimes takes the form of finding ways to overcome our efforts at self-regulation:* Loewenstein, G., & O'Donoghue, T. (2006). "We can do this the easy way or the hard way": Negative emotions, self-regulation, and the law. *The University of Chicago Law Review*, 183-206.
(2) *Neuroimaging approaches could create a product so delicious that all but the most ascetic individuals would find it irresistible*: Ariely, D., & Berns, G. S. (2010). Neuromarketing: The hope and hype of neuroimaging in business. *Nature Reviews Neuroscience*, *11*(4), 0.
(3) *Food marketing may produce far-reaching negative health outcomes*: Harris, J. L., Brownell, K. D., & Bargh, J. A. (2009). The food marketing defense model: Integrating psychological research to protect youth and inform public policy. *Social Issues and Policy Review*, *3*(1), 211-271.

Article in Fast Company: Penenberg, A.L. NeuroFocus uses neuromarketing to hack your brain: Intel, PayPal, Pepsico, Google, HP, Citi, and Microsoft are spending millions to plumb your mind. Fast Company, Aug 8, 2011. Retrieved from:
<http://www.fastcompany.com/1769238/neurofocus-uses-neuromarketing-hack-your-brain>

Habits, the cited definition is by Jonathan van't Riet: van't Riet, J., Sijtsema, S. J., Dagevos, H., & De Bruijn, G. J. (2011). The importance of habits in eating behavior: An overview and recommendations for future research. *Appetite*, *57*(3), 585-596.

Eating is an automatic behavior:
(1) *A review of 'habit'*: Gardner, B. (2014). A review and analysis of the use of 'habit' in understanding, predicting and influencing health-related behaviour. *Health Psychology Review*, Jan 21,1-19.

(2) *Habits proceed without awareness, control, or conscious intent*: Bargh JA. (1994). The four horsemen of automaticity: Awareness, intention, efficiency, and control in social cognition. *Handbook of Social Cognition*, edited by R.S. Wyer and T.K. Srull. (Hillsdale, NJ: Lawrence Erlbaum).
(3) *Consumers repeated their fast food habits, even if they stated intentions to do otherwise*: Ji Song, M., & Wood, W. (2007). Habitual purchase and consumption: Not always what you intend. *Journal of Consumer Psychology*, 17, 261–276.

Under the influence of habits, the brain makes decisions automatically:
(1) *Habits play a large role in unhealthy snacking behavior*: Verhoeven, A. A., Adriaanse, M. A., Evers, C., & de Ridder, D. T. (2012). The power of habits: Unhealthy snacking behaviour is primarily predicted by habit strength. *British Journal of Health Psychology*, *17*(4), 758-770.
(2) Neal, D. T., Wood, W., & Quinn, J. M. (2006). Habits —A repeat performance. *Current Directions in Psychological Science*, *15*(4), 198-202.
(3) *Habitual behavior arises and proceeds unconsciously (mindlessly)*: Aarts, H., Verplanken, B., & Knippenberg, A. (1998). Predicting behavior from actions in the past: Repeated decision making or a matter of habit? *Journal of Applied Social Psychology*, *28*(15), 1355-1374.
(4) *In familiar settings, habitual tendencies override competing intentions:* Gardner, B., de Bruijn, G. J., & Lally, P. (2011). A systematic review and meta-analysis of applications of the self-report habit index to nutrition and physical activity behaviours. *Annals of Behavioral Medicine*, *42*(2), 174-187.

CHAPTER 5. THE ROLE OF CUES IN OVEREATING
Habits are guided by situational cues:
(1) *Habits are cue-contingent, such that the habit-generated impulse will not be activated when the cue is not encountered*: Orbell, S., & Verplanken, B. (2010). The automatic component of habit in health behavior: Habit as cue-contingent automaticity. *Health Psychology*, *29*(4), 374.
(2) *Habitual popcorn eaters at a cinema were minimally influenced by their hunger or how much they liked the food*: Neal, D. T., Wood, W., Wu, M., & Kurlander, D. (2011). The pull of the past: When do habits persist despite

conflict with motives? *Personality and Social Psychology Bulletin*, *37*(11), 1428-1437.

Hyperpalatable food displays are riveting:
(1) *Visually attending to unhealthy food creates a desire to consume the food. To resist the temptation, people have to turn away:* Junghans, A. F., Hooge, I. T., Maas, J., Evers, C., & De Ridder, D. T. (2015). "UnAdulterated—Children and adults' visual attention to healthy and unhealthy food." *Eating Behaviors*, *17*, 90-93.

(2) *Chocolate can involuntarily capture our attention after 100 milliseconds:* Pool, E., Brosch, T., Delplanque, S., & Sander, D. (2014). Where is the chocolate? Rapid spatial orienting toward stimuli associated with primary rewards. *Cognition*, *130*(3), 348-359.

(3) Cohen, D. A., & Babey, S. H. (2012). Contextual influences on eating behaviours: Heuristic processing and dietary choices. *Obesity Reviews*, *13*(9), 766-779.

(4) Cohen, D. A., & Babey, S. H. (2012). Candy at the cash register—A risk factor for obesity and chronic disease. *New England Journal of Medicine*, *367*(15), 1381-1383.

(5) Cohen, D. A. (2008). Neurophysiological pathways to obesity: Below awareness and beyond individual control. *Diabetes*, *57*(7), 1768-1773.

Salience, incentive salience and food cues:
(1) Chandon, P., & Wansink, B. (2011). Is food marketing making us fat? A multi-disciplinary review. *Foundations and Trends® in Marketing*, 5(3), 113-196.

(2) *Incentive salience: Hyperpalatable food cues can trigger intense seeking to obtain and consume the food:* Castro, D. C., & Berridge, K. C. (2014). Advances in the neurobiological bases for food 'liking' versus 'wanting'. *Physiology & Behavior*, *136*, 22-30.

(3) Menzies, J. R., Skibicka, K. P., Egecioglu, E., Leng, G., & Dickson, S. L. (2012). Peripheral signals modifying food reward. *Handbook of Experimental Pharmacology 209*, 131-58.

(4) *Conditioning makes certain food cues overly desirable*: Havermans, R. C. (2013). Pavlovian craving and overeating: A conditioned incentive model. *Current Obesity Reports*, *2*(2), 165-170.

Center for Science in the Public Interest:
(1) Fielding-Singh, P., Almy, J., & Wootan, M.G. Sugar Overload: Retail Checkout Promotes Obesity. Oct. 2014. < http://www.cspinet.org/new/201410161.html> Accessed Feb. 13, 2016.
(2) Almy, J., and Wootan, M.G. (2015) Temptation at checkout: The food industry's sneaky strategy for selling more. Retrieved from < http://cspinet. org/temptationatcheckout/>

Implementation intentions can interrupt automatic responses:
(1) Kroese, F. M., Adriaanse, M. A., Evers, C., & De Ridder, D. T. (2011). Instant success: Turning temptations into cues for goal-directed behavior. *Personality and Social Psychology Bulletin*, 0146167211410889.
(2) *Implementation intentions decreased unhealthy snack consumption*: Adriaanse, M. A., de Ridder, D. T., & de Wit, J. B. (2009). Finding the critical cue: Implementation intentions to change one's diet work best when tailored to personally relevant reasons for unhealthy eating. *Personality and Social Psychology Bulletin*, *35*(1), 60-71.
(3) *Cue-monitoring is a way to gain insight into triggers for unhealthy snacking*: Verhoeven, A. A., Adriaanse, M. A., de Vet, E., Fennis, B. M., & de Ridder, D. T. (2014). Identifying the 'if' for 'if-then' plans: Combining implementation intentions with cue-monitoring targeting unhealthy snacking behaviour. *Psychology & Health*, *29*(12), 1476-1492.
(4) *An if-then plan involves planning out in advance how one wants to deal with willpower challenges*: Gollwitzer, P. M. (2014). Weakness of the will: Is a quick fix possible? *Motivation and Emotion*, *38*(3), 305-322.
(5) *Planning alternative responses to habit cues reduces habitual behaviors*: Adriaanse, M. A., Oettingen, B., Gollwitzer, P. M., Hennes, E. P., de Ridder, D. T. D., & de Wit, J. B. F. (2010). When planning is not enough:

Fighting unhealthy snacking habits by mental contrasting with implementation intentions (MCII). *European Journal of Social Psychology*, *40*, 1277-1293.

Priming, studies by researchers from Yale University: Harris, J. L., Bargh, J. A., & Brownell, K. D. (2009). Priming effects of television food advertising on eating behavior. *Health Psychology*, *28*(4), 404.

Commercials prime consumption:
(1) Kemps, E., Tiggemann, M., & Hollitt, S. (2014). Exposure to television food advertising primes food-related cognitions and triggers motivation to eat. *Psychology & Health*, *29*(10), 1192-1205.
(2) Roberts, M., & Pettigrew, S. (2013). Psychosocial influences on children's food consumption. *Psychology & Marketing*, *30*(2), 103-120.
(3) Bodenlos, J. S., & Wormuth, B. M. (2013). Watching a food-related television show and caloric intake: A laboratory study. *Appetite*, *61*, 8-12.

Unconscious processes explain why willpower often fails: *Strategies include controlling one's exposure to biasing information*: Wilson, T. D., & Brekke, N. (1994). Mental contamination and mental correction: Unwanted influences on judgments and evaluations. *Psychological Bulletin*, *116*(1), 117.

When we are hungry we are more susceptible to cues:
(1) Loewenstein, G. (1996). Out of control: Visceral influences on behavior. *Organizational Behavior and Human Decision Processes*, *65*(3), 272-292.
(2) *Food deprivation increases brain reward activity toward high calorie foods*: Siep, N., Roefs, A., Roebroeck, A., Havermans, R., Bonte, M. L., & Jansen, A. (2009). Hunger is the best spice: An fMRI study of the effects of attention, hunger and calorie content on food reward processing in the amygdala and orbitofrontal cortex. *Behavioural Brain Research*, *198*(1), 149-158.

Hot states, decision making:
(1) Reid, A. Hot-state decision making: Understanding consumer emotion and rationality. Sentient Decision Science, White Paper, Fall 2010.
(2) *Environmental cues may trigger "hot" decision making resulting in impulsive consumption*: Bernheim, B. D., & Rangel, A. (2004). Addiction and cue-triggered decision processes. *American Economic Review*, 1558-1590.
(3) Yang, H., Carmon, Z., Kahn, B., Malani, A., Schwartz, J., Volpp, K., & Wansink, B. (2012). The hot–cold decision triangle: A framework for healthier choices. *Marketing Letters, 23*(2), 457-472.
(4) *When a hot-state is induced through exposure to tempting food, hedonic hunger overrides dieting goals*: Hofmann, W., van Koningsbruggen, G. M., Stroebe, W., Ramanathan, S., & Aarts, H. (2010). As pleasure unfolds: Hedonic responses to tempting food. *Psychological Science 21*, 1863.
(5) Radel, R., & Clément-Guillotin, C. (2012). Evidence of motivational influences in early visual perception: Hunger modulates conscious access. *Psychological Science, 23*(3), 232-234.

If overweight, more susceptible to food cues:
(1) Meyer, M. D., Risbrough, V. B., Liang, J., & Boutelle, K. N. (2015). Pavlovian conditioning to hedonic food cues in overweight and lean individuals. *Appetite, 87*, 56-61.
(2) Ouwehand, C., & Papies, E. K. (2010). Eat it or beat it. The differential effects of food temptations on overweight and normal-weight restrained eaters. *Appetite, 55*(1), 56-60.

Implementation intentions have successfully been used to treat addictive behaviors:
(1) Murgraff, V., White, D., & Phillips, K. (1996). Moderating binge drinking: It is possible to change behaviour if you plan it in advance. *Alcohol and Alcoholism, 31*(6), 577-582.
(2) Armitage, C. J. (2007). Efficacy of a brief worksite intervention to reduce smoking: The roles of behavioral and implementation intentions. *Journal of Occupational Health Psychology, 12*(4), 376.

Marketing Happiness:

(1) Klein, R. Marketing happiness in an unhappy world. Imagination Experience Labs, Nov. 27, 2012. Retrieved from <http://www.imagination. com/en/labs/2012/11/marketing-happiness-unhappy-world>

(2) Casserly, M. (2011). The happiest brands in the world. *Forbes Magazine*, October 6, 2011.

(3) *Marketing fun and happiness to children:* Jenkin, G., Madhvani, N., Signal, L., & Bowers, S. (2014). A systematic review of persuasive marketing techniques to promote food to children on television. *Obesity Reviews, 15*(4), 281-293.

(4) *Nonconscious activation of desirable behavioral states promotes motivation to accomplish these states:* Custers, R., & Aarts, H. (2005). Positive affect as implicit motivator: On the nonconscious operation of behavioral goals. *Journal of Personality and Social Psychology, 89*(2), 129.

(5) *Subliminal smiles altered consumption and desire:* Winkielman, P., Berridge, K. C., & Wilbarger, J. L. (2005). Unconscious affective reactions to masked happy versus angry faces influence consumption behavior and judgments of value. *Personality and Social Psychology Bulletin, 31*(1), 121-135.

(6) *The promise of pleasure is powerful:* Hagtvedt, H., & Patrick, V. M. (2009). The broad embrace of luxury: Hedonic potential as a driver of brand extendibility. *Journal of Consumer Psychology, 19.*

Chocolate ads use thin models (on purpose): Durkin, K., Hendry, A., & Stritzke, W. G. (2013). Mixed selection: Effects of body images, dietary restraint, and persuasive messages on females' orientations towards chocolate. *Appetite, 60,* 95-102.

Food cues subconsciously trigger cravings:

(1) *Pictures of chocolate activate regions of the brain that are involved in drug addiction:* Rolls, E. T., & McCabe, C. (2007). Enhanced affective brain representations of chocolate in cravers vs. non-cravers. *European Journal of Neuroscience, 26*(4), 1067-1076.

(2) *Subliminal conditioning motivates consumers:* Veltkamp, M., Custers, R., & Aarts, H. (2011). Motivating consumer behavior by subliminal conditioning

in the absence of basic needs: Striking even while the iron is cold. *Journal of Consumer Psychology*, 21(1), 49-56.

(3) *Food cravings are triggered by the sight, smell, or imagery of the craved food:* Fedoroff, I. C., Polivy, J., & Herman, C. P. (1997). The effect of pre-exposure to food cues on the eating behavior of restrained and unrestrained eaters. *Appetite*, 28(1), 33-47.

(4) *Even the most fleeting events can motivate us subliminally:* Ziauddeen, H., Subramaniam, N., Gaillard, R., Burke, L. K., Farooqi, I. S., & Fletcher, P. C. (2012). Food images engage subliminal motivation to seek food. *International Journal of Obesity*, 36(9), 1245-1247.

Advertising, addiction metaphor: *The word "addiction" implies devotion, surrendering control, obsessiveness, and preoccupation with the object to the detriment of well-being:*

(1) *Addiction metaphors may legitimize desire by causing us to believe that our wishes are needs:* Belk, R.W., Ger, G., & Askegaard, S. (1996). Metaphors of consumer desire. *Advances in Consumer Research*, Volume 23, edited by K.P. Corfman and J.G. Lynch Jr., pp. 369-373.

(2) *Food manufacturers use addiction terms such as "craving":* Brownell, K. & Gold, M. (2012). Food products. Addiction. Also in the mind [Commentary]. *World Nutrition* 3(9), 392-405.

(3) *A $6 million ad campaign that targeted chocoholics:* Thompson, S. (2003). $6 million effort: Dove targets the chocoholic. *Advertising Age*, 74(37).

(4) *The success of food advertising campaigns might reflect their capacity to manifest cravings:* Johnson, A. W. (2013). Eating beyond metabolic need: How environmental cues influence feeding behavior. *Trends in Neurosciences*, 36(2), 101-109.

The "moment of joy" is momentary:

(1) *When chocolate is consumed as a comfort eating strategy, it is more likely to prolong a bad mood.* Parker, G., Parker, I., & Brotchie, H. (2006). Mood state effects of chocolate. *Journal of Affective Disorders*, 92(2), 149-159.

(2) *Positive affect decreased quickly in those who consumed chocolate:* Hormes, J. M., & Rozin, P. (2011). The temporal dynamics of ambivalence: Changes

in positive and negative affect in relation to consumption of an "emotionally charged" food. *Eating Behaviors, 12*(3), 219-221.
(3) *Consumption accompanied by guilt:* Macht, M., & Dettmer, D. (2006). Everyday mood and emotions after eating a chocolate bar or an apple. *Appetite, 46*(3), 332-336.
(4) *Any positive effect disappeared after 3 minutes:* Macht, M., & Mueller, J. (2007). Immediate effects of chocolate on experimentally induced mood states. *Appetite, 49*(3), 667-674.
(5) *Any pleasure is short lived and accompanied by guilt:* Macdiarmid, J. I., & Hetherington, M. M. (1995). Mood modulation by food: An exploration of affect and cravings in 'chocolate addicts'. *British Journal of Clinical Psychology, 34*(1), 129-138.

It begins to sound like a compulsion:
(1) *Repeated stimulation of reward pathways may lead to neurobiological adaptations that make the intake more compulsive:* Volkow, N. D., & Wise, R. A. (2005). How can drug addiction help us understand obesity? *Nature Neuroscience, 8*(5), 555-560.
(2) *Neuroadaptive responses parallel the shift from motivated to compulsive eating:* Patrono, E., Di Segni, M., Patella, L., Andolina, D., Valzania, A., Latagliata, E. C., ... & Ventura, R. (2015). When chocolate seeking becomes compulsion: Gene-environment interplay. *PLoS One, 10*(3), e0120191.
(3) *Repeated, intermittent intake of palatable food may downregulate reward pathways and amplify stress circuitry, such that continued intake becomes obligatory:* Parylak, S. L., Koob, G. F., & Zorrilla, E. P. (2011). The dark side of food addiction. *Physiology & Behavior, 104*(1), 149-156.
(4) *Refined food addiction is similar to tobacco and alcohol dependence:* Ifland, J. R., Preuss, H. G., Marcus, M. T., Rourke, K. M., Taylor, W. C., Burau, K., ... & Manso, G. (2009). Refined food addiction: A classic substance use disorder. *Medical Hypotheses, 72*(5), 518-526.

Dr. Robert Lustig: Sugar, the most unhappy of pleasures:
(1) Lustig, R. (2009). Sugar: The bitter truth. *University of California Television*. Retrieved from <https://www.youtube.com/watch?v=dBnniua6-oM>

(2) Lustig, R.H. (2013). *Fat Chance: The bitter truth about sugar*. Fourth Estate.
(3) Lustig, RH. The most unhappy of pleasures: This is your brain on sugar. *The Atlantic*, Feb 21, 2012.

Willpower can be eroded by stress and distractions:
(1) *Persistent stress exposure may alter the brain's response to food in ways that pre-dispose individuals to poor eating habits:* Tryon, M. S., Carter, C. S., DeCant, R., & Laugero, K. D. (2013). Chronic stress exposure may affect the brain's response to high calorie food cues and predispose to obesogenic eating habits. *Physiology & Behavior, 120*, 233-242.
(2) Friese, M., Hofmann, W., & Wänke, M. (2008). When impulses take over: Moderated predictive validity of explicit and implicit attitude measures in predicting food choice and consumption behaviour. *British Journal of Social Psychology, 47*(3), 397-419.

Strategy of avoidance is effective:
(1) *Participants inhibited their strong impulses by removing themselves from the tempting stimulus:* Quinn, J. M., Pascoe, A., Wood, W., & Neal, D. T. (2010). Can't control yourself? Monitor those bad habits. *Personality and Social Psychology Bulletin, 36*(4), 499-511.
(2) *By maintaining distance from tempting stimuli and proximity to goal-related stimuli, people increase the likelihood of adhering to their long-term goals:* Fishbach, A., & Shah, J. Y. (2006). Self-control in action: Implicit dispositions toward goals and away from temptations. *Journal of Personality and Social Psychology, 90*(5), 820.
(3) *People with good self-control avoid temptations and problem situations, rather than battling them:* Baumeister, R. Can virtuous habits be cultivated? Big Questions Online, July 24, 2012. Retrieved from <https://www.bigquestionsonline.com/content/can-virtuous-habits-be-cultivated>

Quitting smoking, an example of how avoidance works:
(1) *Smokers experience a heightened nicotine craving when they see smoking cues:* Laibson, D. (2001). A cue-theory of consumption. *The Quarterly Journal of Economics 116*(1), 81-119.

(2) *The ready availability of cigarettes was associated with a 28-fold increase in the odds of smoking*: Shiffman, S., Dunbar, M. S., Li, X., Scholl, S. M., Tindle, H. A., Anderson, S. J., & Ferguson, S. G. (2014). Smoking patterns and stimulus control in intermittent and daily smokers. *PLoS One, 9*(3):e89911.
(3) *Successful quitters remove things from their homes that remind them of smoking*: Sun, X., Prochaska, J. O., Velicer, W. F., & Laforge, R. G. (2007). Transtheoretical principles and processes for quitting smoking: A 24-month comparison of a representative sample of quitters, relapsers, and non-quitters. *Addictive Behaviors, 32*(12), 2707-2726.

Studies by Dr. Molly Crockett:
(1) Crockett, M. J., Braams, B. R., Clark, L., Tobler, P. N., Robbins, T. W., & Kalenscher, T. (2013). Restricting temptations: Neural mechanisms of precommitment. *Neuron, 79*(2), 391-401.
(2) University of Cambridge. (2013). Want to stick with your diet? Better have someone hide the chocolate. Study indicates that removing a temptation is more effective than relying on willpower alone. News Release. Retrieved from <http://www.cam.ac.uk/research/news/want-to-stick-with-your-diet-better-have-someone-hide-the-chocolate>

Dr. Sherry Pagoto: Pagoto, S. Do I have a food addiction? 6 signs of food addiction and 8 steps to overcoming. *Psychology Today*, Web, July 11, 2012. Retrieved from <https://www.psychologytoday.com/blog/shrink/201207/do-i-have-food-addiction>

Your mind will factor in the effort:
(1) Maas, J., de Ridder, D. T., de Vet, E., & De Wit, J. B. (2012). Do distant foods decrease intake? The effect of food accessibility on consumption. *Psychology & Health, 27*(sup2), 59-73.
(2) Privitera, G. J., & Zuraikat, F. M. (2014). Proximity of foods in a competitive food environment influences consumption of a low calorie and a high calorie food. *Appetite, 76*, 175-179.

New, healthy habits can become just as automatic:
(1) *To form a habit, repeat an action consistently in the same context*: Gardner, B., Lally, P., & Wardle, J. (2012). Making health habitual: The psychology of 'habit-formation' and general practice. *British Journal of General Practice, 62*(605), 664-666.
(2) Lally, P., Van Jaarsveld, C. H., Potts, H. W., & Wardle, J. (2010). How are habits formed: Modelling habit formation in the real world. *European Journal of Social Psychology, 40*(6), 998-1009.
(3) *Behavior change was initially experienced as effortful, but as automaticity increased, enactment became easier*: Lally, P., Wardle, J., & Gardner, B. (2011). Experiences of habit formation: A qualitative study. *Psychology, Health & Medicine, 16*(4), 484-489.

CHAPTER 6. EAT MINDFULLY
Making the unconscious conscious: *Mindfulness (Review):* Keng, S. L., Smoski, M. J., & Robins, C. J. (2011). Effects of mindfulness on psychological health: A review of empirical studies. *Clinical Psychology Review, 31*(6), 1041-1056.

Dr. Ellen Langer:
(1) *Dr. Langer says that "No one gains 10 pounds overnight"*: The Diane Rehm Show. (2014). An interview with Ellen Langer: Mindfulness and the power of thought. Dec 1, 2014.
(2) Langer E.J. (2014). *Mindfulness, 25th Anniversary Edition* (A Merloyd Lawrence Book). Da Capo Press.

Wherever You Go, There You Are: Kabat-Zinn, J. (1994). *Wherever you go, there you are: Mindfulness meditation in everyday life*. Hyperion.

Five facets of mindfulness:
(1) Baer, R. A., Smith, G. T., Lykins, E., Button, D., Krietemeyer, J., Sauer, S., ... & Williams, J. M. G. (2008). Construct validity of the five

facet mindfulness questionnaire in meditating and nonmeditating samples. *Assessment*, *15*(3), 329-342.
(2) Spears, C. A., Houchins, S. C., Stewart, D. W., Chen, M., Correa-Fernández, V., Cano, M. Á., ... & Wetter, D. W. (2015). Nonjudging facet of mindfulness predicts enhanced smoking cessation in Hispanics. *Psychology of Addictive Behaviors*, *29*(4), 918.

Mindfulness training is being used in treatment programs:
(1) Garland, E. L., Boettiger, C. A., Gaylord, S., Chanon, V. W., & Howard, M. O. (2012). Mindfulness is inversely associated with alcohol attentional bias among recovering alcohol-dependent adults. *Cognitive Therapy and Research*, *36*(5), 441-450.
(2) Garland, E. L., Roberts-Lewis, A., Kelley, K., Tronnier, C., & Hanley, A. (2014). Cognitive and affective mechanisms linking trait mindfulness to craving among individuals in addiction recovery. *Substance Use & Misuse*, *49*(5), 525-535.
(3) Garland, E. L., Froeliger, B., & Howard, M. O. (2013). Mindfulness training targets neurocognitive mechanisms of addiction at the attention-appraisal-emotion interface. *Frontiers in Psychiatry*, *4*, 173.
(4) Wenk-Sormaz, H. (2005). Meditation can reduce habitual responding. *Advances in Mind-Body Medicine*, *21*(3-4), 33-49.
(5) Brewer, J. A., Elwafi, H. M., & Davis, J. H. (2013). Craving to quit: Psychological models and neurobiological mechanisms of mindfulness training as treatment for addictions. *Psychology of Addictive Behaviors*, *27*(2), 366.
(6) Hölzel, B. K., Carmody, J., Vangel, M., Congleton, C., Yerramsetti, S. M., Gard, T., & Lazar, S. W. (2011). Mindfulness practice leads to increases in regional brain gray matter density. *Psychiatry Research: Neuroimaging*, *191*(1), 36-43.

Mindfulness counteracts mindless eating, boosts weight loss:
(1) O'Reilly, G. A., Cook, L., Spruijt-Metz, D., & Black, D. S. (2014). Mindfulness-based interventions for obesity-related eating behaviours: A literature review. *Obesity Reviews*, *15*(6), 453-461.

(2) Kristeller, J., Wolever, R. Q., & Sheets, V. (2014). Mindfulness-based eating awareness training (MB-EAT) for binge eating: A randomized clinical trial. *Mindfulness*, 5(3), 282-297.
(3) Bahl, S., Milne, G. R., Ross, S. M., & Chan, K. (2013). Mindfulness: A long-term solution for mindless eating by college students. *Journal of Public Policy & Marketing*, 32(2), 173-184.

Acting with awareness, non-judging: The nonjudgmental awareness of experiences in the present moment reduces distress and promotes well-being:
(1) Hölzel, B. K., Lazar, S. W., Gard, T., Schuman-Olivier, Z., Vago, D. R., & Ott, U. (2011). How does mindfulness meditation work? Proposing mechanisms of action from a conceptual and neural perspective. *Perspectives on Psychological Science*, 6(6), 537-559.
(2) *The ability to describe and accept experiences may buffer the impact of psychological distress:* Daubenmier J., Hayden, D., Chang, V., & Epel, E. (2014). It's not what you think, it's how you relate to it: Dispositional mindfulness moderates the relationship between psychological distress and the cortisol awakening response. *Psychoneuroendocrinology, 48*, 11-18.

Observing: Papies, E. K., Pronk, T. M., Keesman, M., & Barsalou, L. W. (2015). The benefits of simply observing: Mindful attention modulates the link between motivation and behavior. *Journal of Personality and Social Psychology*, 108(1), 148-170.

Describing: *Putting feelings into words helps people deal with negative emotions*: Lieberman, M. D., Eisenberger, N. I., Crockett, M. J., Tom, S. M., Pfeifer, J. H., & Way, B. M. (2007). Putting feelings into words affect labeling disrupts amygdala activity in response to affective stimuli. *Psychological Science, 18*(5), 421-428.

Disrupting automatic reactions to cravings (Set a timer for 20 minutes):
(1) *In a survey of over 200 people in everyday life, the median experienced duration of desires was 16–20 minutes*: Hofmann, W., Baumeister, R. F., Förster, G., & Vohs, K. D. (2012). Everyday temptations: An experience sampling

study of desire, conflict, and self-control. *Journal of Personality and Social Psychology, 102*(6), 1318.

(2) Mead, N.L., & Patrick, V.M. In praise of putting things off: Postponing consumption pleasures facilitates self-control. (2011). *Advances in Consumer Research, 39,* 30-31.

(3) *Postponement keeps the temptation at arm's length and encourages self-control:* Pappas, S. (2012). To resist temptation, put it off. *Live Science,* Jan 30, 2012. Retrieved from <http://www.livescience.com/18199-postponement-resist-temptation.html>

(4) *Postponing consumption to an unspecified future time reduced the consumption of, an unhealthy snack. This strategy works by reducing desire:* SPSP News Center. Willpower and desires: Turning up the volume on what you want most. (2012). Annual Meeting of the Society for Personality and Social Psychology. Retrieved from <http://www.spsp.org/news-center/press-releases/willpower-and-desires-turning-volume-what-you-want-most>

(5) *Adopt the goal to be inactive in the face of temptation:* Hepler, J., Albarracin, D., McCulloch, K. C., & Noguchi, K. (2012). Being active and impulsive: The role of goals for action and inaction in self-control. *Motivation and Emotion, 36*(4), 416-424.

Eating often occurs mindlessly. Mindfulness counters automatic behaviors:
(1) *Enhanced attention to present experiences can strengthen the link between intentions and behavior:* Chatzisarantis, N. L., & Hagger, M. S. (2007). Mindfulness and the intention-behavior relationship within the theory of planned behavior. *Personality and Social Psychology Bulletin, 33*(5), 663-676.

(2) *Women with higher mindfulness scores were less likely to be overweight:* Camilleri, G. M., Méjean, C., Bellisle, F., Hercberg, S., & Péneau, S. (2015). Association between mindfulness and weight status in a general population from the NutriNet-Santé study. *PloS One, 10*(6), e0127447.

(3) *Once habits are monitored, the agent can override them. The most important part of this is simply the monitoring:* Dill, B., & Holton, R. (2014). The addict in us all. *Frontiers in Psychiatry, 5,* 139.

In order to make the unconscious conscious, I kept a detailed journal: Writing
in a journal increases weight loss: Kon, A., Beresford, S. A., Alfano, C. M.,
Foster-Schubert, K. E., Neuhouser, M. L., Johnson, D. B., ... & McTiernan,
A. (2012). Self-monitoring and eating-related behaviors are associated with
12-month weight loss in postmenopausal overweight-to-obese women.
Journal of the Academy of Nutrition and Dietetics, 112(9), 1428-1435.

Discovering automatic habit loops: Duhigg, Charles (2012). *The power of
habit: Why we do what we do in life and business.* New York: Random House.

Rumination and comfort eating:
(1) *Comfort eaters preferentially consume sweet, fatty, energy-dense food*: Gibson,
E. L. (2012). The psychobiology of comfort eating: Implications for neu-
ropharmacological interventions. *Behavioural Pharmacology, 23*(5 and 6),
442-460.
(2) Schepers, R., & Markus, C. R. (2015). Gene × cognition interaction on
stress-induced eating: Effect of rumination. *Psychoneuroendocrinology, 54,*
41-53

Emotional eating is a reason why many weight-loss plans fail:
(1) *There is a direct connection between emotional eating and BMI. A reduced
frequency of emotional eating was associated with greater weight loss*: Blair, A. J.,
Lewis, V. J., & Booth, D. A. (1990). Does emotional eating interfere with
success in attempts at weight control?. *Appetite, 15*(2), 151-157.
(2) *Negative mood sensitizes the brain's reward system to hyperpalatable food cues,
thereby precipitating self-regulatory failure and, in turn, overeating*: Wagner,
D. D., Boswell, R. G., Kelley, W. M., & Heatherton, T. F. (2012). Inducing
negative affect increases the reward value of appetizing foods in dieters.
Journal of Cognitive Neuroscience, 24(7), 1625-1633.
(3) Crockett, A. C., Myhre, S. K., & Rokke, P. D. (2015). Boredom prone-
ness and emotion regulation predict emotional eating. *Journal of Health
Psychology, 20*(5), 670-680.
(4) Singh, M. (2014). Mood, food, and obesity. *Frontiers in Psychology, 5*:925.

Cognitive defusion is an effective way of dealing with negative emotions:
(1) Teasdale, J. D., Moore, R. G., Hayhurst, H., Pope, M., Williams, S., & Segal, Z. V. (2002). Metacognitive awareness and prevention of relapse in depression: Empirical evidence. *Journal of Consulting and Clinical Psychology*, *70*(2), 275.
(2) Niemeier, H. M., Leahey, T., Reed, K. P., Brown, R. A., & Wing, R. R. (2012). An acceptance-based behavioral intervention for weight loss: A pilot study. *Behavior Therapy*, *43*(2), 427-435.
(3) Forman, E. M., & Butryn, M. L. (2015). A new look at the science of weight control: How acceptance and commitment strategies can address the challenge of self-regulation. *Appetite*, *84*, 171-180.
(4) Armitage, C. J. (2015). Randomized test of a brief psychological intervention to reduce and prevent emotional eating in a community sample. *Journal of Public Health*, *37*(3), 438-444.
(5) Frewen, P. A., Evans, E. M., Maraj, N., Dozois, D. J., & Partridge, K. (2008). Letting go: Mindfulness and negative automatic thinking. *Cognitive Therapy and Research*, *32*(6), 758-774.

Participants who were taught to "step back" from their cravings ate less chocolate: Jenkins, K. T., & Tapper, K. (2014). Resisting chocolate temptation using a brief mindfulness strategy. *British Journal of Health Psychology*, *19*(3), 509-522.

The advantages of non-reactivity: Dr. Lucie Hemmen: Hemmen, L. (2012). Teen girls and the practice of non-reactivity. Tips for keeping your cool with your teenager. *Psychology Today*, July 31, 2012.

Cravings that seem to dominate our attention will fade away: Alberts, H. J. E. M., Thewissen, R., & Raes, L. (2012). Dealing with problematic eating behavior: The effects of a mindfulness-based intervention on eating behaviour, food cravings, dichotomous thinking and body image concern. *Appetite*, *58*(3), 847-851.

Rumination is associated with unhappiness:
(1) *The default mode of humans appears to be that of mind-wandering, which correlates with unhappiness. Meditation decreases mind-wandering:* Brewer, J. A., Worhunsky, P. D., Gray, J. R., Tang, Y. Y., Weber, J., & Kober, H. (2011). Meditation experience is associated with differences in default mode network activity and connectivity. *Proceedings of the National Academy of Sciences, 108*(50), 20254-20259.
(2) Smallwood, J., & O' Connor, R. C. (2011). Imprisoned by the past: Unhappy moods lead to a retrospective bias to mind wandering. *Cognition & Emotion, 25*(8), 1481-1490.

Mindfulness has a (positive) ripple effect:
(1) Brown, K. W., & Ryan, R. M. (2003). The benefits of being present: Mindfulness and its role in psychological well-being. *Journal of Personality and Social Psychology, 84*(4), 822.
(2) Garland, E. L., Geschwind, N., Peeters, F., & Wichers, M. (2015). Mindfulness training promotes upward spirals of positive affect and cognition: Multilevel and autoregressive latent trajectory modeling analyses. *Frontiers in Psychology, 6*, 15.
(3) Desbordes, G., Gard, T., Hoge, E. A., Hölzel, B. K., Kerr, C., Lazar, S. W., ... & Vago, D. R. (2014). Moving beyond mindfulness: Defining equanimity as an outcome measure in meditation and contemplative research. *Mindfulness, 6*(2), 356-372.
(4) *Mindfulness can help to reduce automatic negative self-evaluations, increase tolerance for negative affect, and engender self-compassion and empathy:* Farb, N. A., Anderson, A. K., & Segal, Z. V. (2012). The mindful brain and emotion regulation in mood disorders. *Canadian Journal of Psychiatry, 57*(2), 70.
(5) *Mindfulness enables positive reappraisal of stressful events. Positive reappraisal is the extent one copes with adverse life events with thoughts such as "I think I can learn something from the situation":* Garland, E., Gaylord, S., & Park, J. (2009). The role of mindfulness in positive reappraisal. *Explore: The Journal of Science and Healing, 5*(1), 37-44.

(6) Mindfulness can facilitate well-being by adding clarity and vividness to current experience and encouraging moment-to-moment sensory contact with life: Brown, K. W., Ryan, R. M., & Creswell, J. D. (2007). Mindfulness: Theoretical foundations and evidence for its salutary effects. *Psychological inquiry*, *18*(4), 211-237.

CHAPTER 7. VISUALIZE YOUR GOAL
Rosabeth Moss Kanter: Harvard Business School. (2001). What Makes a Good Leader. Retrieved from <https://www.alumni.hbs.edu/stories/Pages/story-bulletin.aspx?num=3059>

Visualization, athletes: Ungerleider, S. (2005). *Mental training for peak performance: Top athletes reveal the mind exercises they use to excel.* New York: Rodale Inc.

Visualization increases motivation, concentration, and goal attainment:
(1) Taylor, S. E., Pham, L. B., Rivkin, I. D., & Armor, D. A. (1998). Harnessing the imagination: Mental simulation, self-regulation, and coping. *American Psychologist, 53*(4), 429.
(2) *Episodic simulation of future events involves drawing on elements of past experiences in order to envisage and mentally "try out" one or more versions of what might happen*: Schacter, D. L., Addis, D. R., & Buckner, R. L. (2008). Episodic simulation of future events. *Annals of the New York Academy of Sciences, 1124*(1), 39-60.
(3) Oettingen, G., Hönig, G., & Gollwitzer, P. M. (2000). Effective self-regulation of goal attainment. *International Journal of Educational Research, 33*(7), 705-732.
(4) *Whether a goal is activated by conscious or nonconscious means, the goal will guide a person's behavior from that point on*: Bargh, J. A., Gollwitzer, P. M., Lee-Chai, A., Barndollar, K., & Trötschel, R. (2001). The automated will: Nonconscious activation and pursuit of behavioral goals. *Journal of Personality and Social Psychology, 81*(6), 1014.
(5) *Highly developed mental imagery leads to more effective, specific intentions and better goal achievement*: Knäuper, B., Roseman, M., Johnson, P. J., &

Krantz, L. H. (2009). Using mental imagery to enhance the effectiveness of implementation intentions. *Current Psychology*, *28*(3), 181-186.

Visualization can boost weight loss: Hattar, A., Hagger, M. S., & Pal, S. (2015). Weight-loss intervention using implementation intentions and mental imagery: a randomized control trial study protocol. *BMC Public Health*, *15*(1), 196.

Mental contrasting, comparing one's present reality with a goal:
(1) *One way of enhancing self-regulatory success is to increase self-awareness of the discrepancy between one's current state and a particular standard towards which the individual aspires:* Pychyl, T.A. Awareness: A key piece in the procrastination puzzle. *Psychology Today* blog, Dec. 7, 2011.
(2) Johannessen, K. B., Oettingen, G., & Mayer, D. (2012). Mental contrasting of a dieting wish improves self-reported health behaviour. *Psychology & Health*, *27*(sup2), 43-58.
(3) Amin, A. (2014). Why does mental contrasting work? Happier Human (web). Retrieved from <http://happierhuman.com/mental-contrasting/#Why_Does_Mental_Contrasting_Work> (4) *While solely fantasizing about a desired future leads to little behavior change, mental contrasting leads to skilled problem solving and substantial behavior change:* Oettingen, G., and Schwörer, B. (2013). Mind wandering via mental contrasting as a tool for behavior change. *Frontiers in Psychology*, *4*, 562.

The power of vividly imagining the future:
(1) Suddendorf, T., & Corballis, M. C. (2007). The evolution of foresight: What is mental time travel, and is it unique to humans? *Behavioral and Brain Sciences*, *30*(03), 299-313 (also see discussion on pages 313-51.)
(2) *Episodic future thinking involves projecting the self into the future to pre-experience an event*: Atance, C. M., & O'Neill, D. K. (2001). Episodic future thinking. *Trends in Cognitive Sciences*, *5*(12), 533-539.
(3) Lyman, B., Bernardin, S., & Thomas, S. (1980). Frequency of imagery in emotional experience. *Perceptual and Motor Skills*, *50*(3c), 1159-1162.

Those who visualized themselves in the future, as if it were happening today, consumed fewer calories:
(1) Daniel, T. O., Stanton, C. M., & Epstein, L. H. (2013). The future is now: Reducing impulsivity and energy intake using episodic future thinking. *Psychological Science*, 24(11):2339-42.
(2) *Visualization of the future improved the ability of lean and obese individuals to delay gratification*: Daniel, T. O., Stanton, C. M., & Epstein, L. H. (2013). The future is now: Comparing the effect of episodic future thinking on impulsivity in lean and obese individuals. Appetite, 71, 120-125.
(3) Sze, Y. Y., Daniel, T. O., Kilanowski, C. K., Collins, R. L., & Epstein, L. H. (2015). Web-based and mobile delivery of an episodic future thinking intervention for overweight and obese families: A feasibility study. *JMIR mHealth and uHealth*, 3(4).

Wray Herbert: Herbert, W. (2013). For obesity, the future is now. Association for Psychological Science, April 12, 2013. Retrieved from <http://www.psychologicalscience.org/index.php/news/were-only-human/for-obesity-the-future-is-now.html>

CHAPTER 8. DOCUMENT YOUR JOURNEY
Julia Cameron: "Writing is a weight-loss tool: overlooked, underused, and extremely powerful." In: Cameron, J. (2007). *The writing diet: Write yourself right-size*. New York: Penguin.

Journaling as a simple yet powerful tool:
(1) Cameron, L. D., & Nicholls, G. (1998). Expression of stressful experiences through writing: Effects of a self-regulation manipulation for pessimists and optimists. *Health Psychology*, 17(1), 84.
(2) Baker, R. C., & Kirschenbaum, D. S. (1998). Weight control during the holidays: Highly consistent self-monitoring as a potentially useful coping mechanism. *Health Psychology*, 17(4), 367.
(3) Quinn, J. M., Pascoe, A., Wood, W., & Neal, D. T. (2010). Can't control yourself? Monitor those bad habits. *Personality and Social Psychology Bulletin*, 36(4), 499-511.

Self-monitoring is important for weight loss success:
(1) Kong, A., Beresford, S. A., Alfano, C. M., Foster-Schubert, K. E., Neuhouser, M. L., Johnson, D. B., ... & McTiernan, A. (2012). Self-monitoring and eating-related behaviors are associated with 12-month weight loss in postmenopausal overweight-to-obese women. *Journal of the Academy of Nutrition and Dietetics, 112*(9), 1428-1435.
(2) *Daily self-monitoring of weight, physical activity, and fruit/vegetable consumption is an effective approach for maintaining weight loss*: Akers, J. D., Cornett, R. A., Savla, J. S., Davy, K. P., & Davy, B. M. (2012). Daily self-monitoring of body weight, step count, fruit/vegetable intake, and water consumption: A feasible and effective long-term weight loss maintenance approach. *Journal of the Academy of Nutrition and Dietetics, 112*(5), 685-692.
(3) *The combination of high frequency* plus *high consistency of dietary self-monitoring improves long-term success in weight management*: Peterson, N. D., Middleton, K. R., Nackers, L. M., Medina, K. E., Milsom, V. A., & Perri, M. G. (2014). Dietary self-monitoring and long-term success with weight management. *Obesity, 22*(9), 1962-1967.
(4) *Self-monitoring was part of 92% of successful weight-loss interventions*: Ramage, S., Farmer, A., Apps Eccles, K., & McCargar, L. (2013). Healthy strategies for successful weight loss and weight maintenance: A systematic review. Applied Physiology, Nutrition, and Metabolism, 39(1), 1-20.

Self-weighing boosts weight loss:
(1) Steinberg, D. M., Bennett, G. G., Askew, S., & Tate, D. F. (2015). Weighing every day matters: Daily weighing improves weight loss and adoption of weight control behaviors. *Journal of the Academy of Nutrition and Dietetics, 115*(4), 511-518.
(2) *Consistent self-weighing may help individuals maintain their successful weight loss by allowing them to catch weight gains before they escalate and make behavior changes to prevent additional weight gain*: Butryn, M. L., Phelan, S., Hill, J. O., & Wing, R. R. (2007). Consistent self-monitoring of weight: a key component of successful weight loss maintenance. *Obesity, 15*(12), 3091-3096.

A change of habit can take 66 to 250 repetitions of the new behavior: Lally, P., Van Jaarsveld, C. H., Potts, H. W., & Wardle, J. (2010). How are habits formed: Modelling habit formation in the real world. *European Journal of Social Psychology, 40*(6), 998-1009.

Monitoring the process of habit formation: Hennecke, M., & Freund, A. M. (2014). Identifying success on the process level reduces negative effects of prior weight loss on subsequent weight loss during a low-calorie diet. *Applied Psychology: Health and Well-Being, 6*(1), 48-66.

CHAPTER 9. PRACTICE COMPASSION
Subconscious scripts can keep us stuck:
(1) *Perfectionism is associated with psychological distress:* Flett, G.L., Hewitt, P.L., Blankstein, K.R., & Gray, L. (1998). Psychological distress and the frequency of perfectionistic thinking. *Journal of Personality and Social Psychology, 75*(5), 1363-81.
(2) *Binge eaters suffer from high perceived expectations:* Heatherton, T. F., & Baumeister, R. F. (1991). Binge eating as escape from self-awareness. *Psychological Bulletin, 110*(1), 86.

Many therapies use metacognition to overcome negative self-thinking: Verplanken, B., Friborg, O., Wang, C. E., Trafimow, D., & Woolf, K. (2007). Mental habits: Metacognitive reflection on negative self-thinking. *Journal of Personality and Social Psychology, 92*(3), 526.

Self-talk can be helpful or detrimental:
(1) Schwartz, R. M. (1986). The internal dialogue: On the asymmetry between positive and negative coping thoughts. *Cognitive Therapy and Research, 10*(6), 591-605.
(2) Schwartz, R. M., & Caramoni, G. L. (1989). Cognitive balance and psychopathology: Evaluation of an information processing model of positive and negative states of mind. *Clinical Psychology Review, 9*(3), 271-294.

(3) Conversano, C., Rotondo, A., Lensi, E., Della Vista, O., Arpone, F., & Reda, M. A. (2010). Optimism and its impact on mental and physical well-being. *Clinical Practice and Epidemiology in Mental Health: CP & EMH, 6*, 25.

Cognitive distortions contribute to overeating, diet failure:
(1) Özdel, K., Taymur, I., Guriz, S. O., Tulaci, R. G., Kuru, E., & Turkcapar, M. H. (2014). Measuring cognitive errors using the Cognitive Distortions Scale (CDS): Psychometric properties in clinical and non-clinical samples. *PLoS One, 9*(8), e105956.
(2) *A dichotomous (black-and-white) thinking style was more common in women who regained the weight they had lost:* Byrne, S., Cooper, Z., & Fairburn, C. (2003). Weight maintenance and relapse in obesity: A qualitative study. *International Journal of Obesity, 27*(8), 955-962.
(3) *An all-or-nothing approach (rigid cognitive restraint) decreases the chance of weight loss:* Teixeira, P. J., Silva, M. N., Coutinho, S. R., Palmeira, A. L., Mata, J., Vieira, P. N., ... & Sardinha, L. B. (2010). Mediators of weight loss and weight loss maintenance in middle-aged women. *Obesity, 18*(4), 725-735.
(4) *All-or-nothing thinking is the basis* for *perfectionism:* Sherry, S. B., Sabourin, B. C., Hall, P. A., Hewitt, P. L., Flett, G. L., & Gralnick, T. M. (2014). The perfectionism model of binge eating: Testing unique contributions, mediating mechanisms, and cross-cultural similarities using a daily diary methodology. *Psychology of Addictive Behaviors, 28*(4), 1230.

Dr. David Burns:
(1) Burns, David D. (1999). *The feeling good handbook.* New York: Plume.
(2) Burns, David D., M.D. (1980). *Feeling good: The new mood therapy.* New York: Avon Books.

What-the-hell effect: A common pattern for addicts and chronic dieters when they "fall off the wagon": Heatherton, T. F., & Wagner, D. D. (2011). Cognitive neuroscience of self-regulation failure. *Trends in Cognitive Sciences, 15*(3), 132-139.

Dr. Kristin Neff: Neff, Kristin, Ph.D. (2011). *Self-Compassion: The proven power of being kind to yourself.* New York: HarperCollins.

Three aspects of self-compassion: Neff, K. (2003). Self-compassion: An alternative conceptualization of a healthy attitude toward oneself. *Self and Identity,* 2(2), 85-101.

Positive effects of self-compassion:
(1) Neff, K. (2015). The physiology of self-compassion. Retrieved from <http://self-compassion.org/the-physiology-of-self-compassion/>
(2) Leary, M. R., Tate, E. B., Adams, C. E., Allen, A. B., & Hancock, J. (2007). Self–compassion and reactions to unpleasant self–relevant events: The implications of treating oneself kindly. *Journal of Personality and Social Psychology, 92,* 887–904.
(3) *Self-compassion is an important predictor of psychological health:* Van Dam, N. T., Sheppard, S. C., Forsyth, J. P., & Earleywine, M. (2011). Self-compassion is a better predictor than mindfulness of symptom severity and quality of life in mixed anxiety and depression. *Journal of anxiety Disorders,* 25(1), 123-130.
(4) Sheldon, K. M., & Lyubomirsky, S. (2006). How to increase and sustain positive emotion: The effects of expressing gratitude and visualizing best possible selves. *The Journal of Positive Psychology,* 1(2), 73-82.
(5) *People can increase their happiness through simple intentional positive activities, such as expressing gratitude or practicing kindness:* Lyubomirsky, S., & Layous, K. (2013). How do simple positive activities increase well-being?. *Current Directions in Psychological Science,* 22(1), 57-62.

Journaling (self-monitoring) promotes mindfulness and self-compassion:
The keeping of diaries that focus on how one is eating promotes long-term weight loss. Journaling should be done in a self-compassionate (non-judgmental) way: Mantzios, M., and Wilson, J. C. (2014). Making concrete construals mindful: A novel approach for developing mindfulness and self-compassion to assist weight loss. *Psychology & Health,* 29(4), 422-441.

Self-compassion boosts weight loss and self-control:
(1) *A mindfulness plus self-compassion group lost more weight:* Mantzios, M., & Wilson, J. C. (2014). Exploring mindfulness and mindfulness with self-compassion-centered interventions to assist weight loss: Theoretical considerations and preliminary results of a randomized pilot study. *Mindfulness,* July 2014, 1-12.
(2) Sirois, F. M. (2015). A self-regulation resource model of self-compassion and health behavior intentions in emerging adults. *Preventive Medicine Reports, 2,* 218-222.
(3) Terry, M. L., and Leary, M. R. (2011). Self-compassion, self-regulation, and health. *Self and Identity, 10*(3), 352-362.
(4) *Self-control is improved when people acknowledge and accept their errors:* Inzlicht, M., Legault, L., & Teper, R. (2014). Exploring the mechanisms of self-control improvement. *Current Directions in Psychological Science, 23*(4), 302-307.
(5) *Self–compassion modulates the "what-the-hell" effect:* Adams, C. E., & Leary, M. R. (2007). Promoting self-compassionate attitudes toward eating among restrictive and guilty eaters. *Journal of Social and Clinical Psychology, 26*(10), 1120-1144.

Positive thoughts and emotions lead to positive behaviors:
(1) Burns, A. B., Brown, J. S., Sachs-Ericsson, N., Plant, E. A., Curtis, J. T., Fredrickson, B. L., & Joiner, T. E. (2008). Upward spirals of positive emotion and coping: Replication, extension, and initial exploration of neurochemical substrates. *Personality and Individual Differences, 44*(2), 360-370.
(2) Wright, J., & Mischel, W. (1982). Influence of affect on cognitive social learning person variables. *Journal of Personality and Social Psychology, 43*(5), 901.
(3) *Positive mood enhances self-efficacy, despondent mood diminishes it:* Bandura, A. (1989). Regulation of cognitive processes through perceived self-efficacy. *Developmental Psychology, 25*(5), 729.
(4) Seppala, E. (2013). The compassionate mind: Science shows why it's health and how it spreads. *APS Observer, 26,* 5.
(5) *Positive moods increase the salience of long-term goals, leading to greater preference for healthy foods over indulgent foods:* Gardner, M. P., Wansink, B., Kim,

J., & Park, S. B. (2014). Better moods for better eating? How mood influences food choice. *J Consumer Psychol*, *24*, 320-335.

According to a recent article in Scientific American: Ricard, M., Lutz, A., & Davidson, R. J. (2014). Mind of the Meditator. *Scientific American*, *311*(5), 38-45.

CHAPTER 10. REDUCE STRESS
People who are stressed often cope by engaging in unhealthy behaviors:
(1) Sinha, R., & Jastreboff, A. M. (2013). Stress as a common risk factor for obesity and addiction. *Biological Psychiatry*, *73*(9), 827-835.
(2) Stambor, Z. (2006). Stressed out nation: Many Americans resort to unhealthy habits to help manage extreme stress, a new survey suggests. *Monitor on Psychology*, *37*(4), 28.
(3) Goeders, N. E. (2003). The impact of stress on addiction. *European Neuropsychopharmacology*, *13*(6), 435-441.
(4) Taylor S. B., Anglin, J. M., Paode, P. R., Riggert, A. G., Olive, M. F., & Conrad, C. D. (2014). Chronic stress may facilitate the recruitment of habit-and addiction-related neurocircuitries through neuronal restructuring of the striatum. *Neuroscience*, *280*, 231-242.
(5) Arnsten, A. F. (2009). Stress signalling pathways that impair prefrontal cortex structure and function. *Nature Reviews Neuroscience*, *10*(6), 410-422.
(6) Aschbacher, K., Kornfeld, S., Picard, M., Puterman, E., Havel, P. J., Stanhope, K., ... & Epel, E. (2014). Chronic stress increases vulnerability to diet-related abdominal fat, oxidative stress, and metabolic risk. *Psychoneuroendocrinology*, *46*, 14-22.

Chronic stress is associated with a greater desire for hyperpalatable foods
(1) *Stress promotes hedonic eating:* Epel, E. S., Tomiyama, A. J., & Dallman, M. F. (2012). Stress and reward neural networks, eating, and obesity. *Food and Addiction: A Comprehensive Handbook. New York: Oxford University Press. (Laraia).*
(2) *Chronic stress has a direct effect on food cravings, and food cravings have a direct effect on body mass index*: Chao, A., Grilo, C. M., White, M. A., &

Sinha, R. (2015). Food cravings mediate the relationship between chronic stress and body mass index. *Journal of Health Psychology*, 20(6), 721-729.
(3) Pool, E., Brosch, T., Delplanque, S., & Sander, D. (2015). Stress increases cue-triggered 'wanting' for sweet reward in humans. *Journal of Experimental Psychology: Animal Learning and Cognition*, 41(2), 128.
(4) Tryon, M. S., Carter, C. S., DeCant, R., & Laugero, K. D. (2013). Chronic stress exposure may affect the brain's response to high calorie food cues and predispose to obesogenic eating habits. *Physiology & Behavior*, 120, 233-242.
(5) *Eating sugar may quiet stress signals in the brain, leading some people to seek comfort by consuming more sweets*: Tryon, M. S., Stanhope, K. L., Epel, E. S., Mason, A. E., Brown, R., Medici, V., ... & Laugero, K. D. (2015). Excessive sugar consumption may be a difficult habit to break: A view from the brain and body. *The Journal of Clinical Endocrinology & Metabolism*, jc-2014.
(6) Roberts, C. J., Campbell, I. C., & Troop, N. (2014). Increases in weight during chronic stress are partially associated with a switch in food choice towards increased carbohydrate and saturated fat intake. *European Eating Disorders Review*, 22(1), 77-82.

Proven stress relievers:
(1) Albers, Susan, PSY.D. (2009). *50 ways to soothe yourself without food.* Oakland, CA: New Harbinger Publications, Inc.
(2) *Contact with nature*: Capaldi, C. A., Dopko, R. L., & Zelenski, J. M. (2014). The relationship between nature connectedness and happiness: A meta-analysis. *Frontiers in Psychology*, 5, 976.
(3) *Yoga*: Gard, T., Noggle, J. J., Park, C. L., Vago, D. R., & Wilson, A. (2014). Potential self-regulatory mechanisms of yoga for psychological health. *Frontiers in Human Neuroscience*, 8, 770.
(4) *Yoga*: Li, A. W., & Goldsmith, C. A. (2012). The effects of yoga on anxiety and stress. *Altern Med Rev*, 17(1), 21-35.
(5) *Exercise*: Hogan, C. L., Mata, J., & Carstensen, L. L. (2013). Exercise holds immediate benefits for affect and cognition in younger and older adults. *Psychology and Aging*, 28(2), 587.

(6) *An acute exercise bout (20 minutes) positively impacts well-being:* Kopp, M., Steinlechner, M., Ruedl, G., Ledochowski, L., Rumpold, G., & Taylor, A. H. (2012). Acute effects of brisk walking on affect and psychological well-being in individuals with type 2 diabetes. *Diabetes Research and Clinical Practice, 95*(1), 25-29.

(7) *Music:* Linnemann, A., Ditzen, B., Strahler, J., Doerr, J. M., & Nater, U. M. (2015). Music listening as a means of stress reduction in daily life. *Psychoneuroendocrinology, 60,* 82-90.

(8) *Mindfulness-based stress reduction:* Nyklíček, I., & Kuijpers, K. F. (2008). Effects of mindfulness-based stress reduction intervention on psychological well-being and quality of life: Is increased mindfulness indeed the mechanism? *Annals of Behavioral Medicine, 35*(3), 331-340.

Women who experienced the greatest reduction in stress had the most loss of abdominal fat: Daubenmier, J., Kristeller, J., Hecht, F. M., Maninger, N., Kuwata, M., Jhaveri, K., ... & Epel, E. (2011). Mindfulness intervention for stress eating to reduce cortisol and abdominal fat among overweight and obese women: An exploratory randomized controlled study. *Journal of Obesity, 2011,* Article ID 651936.

Deep breathing counters the effects of stress, builds self-control:
(1) McCraty, R., & Shaffer, F. (2015). Heart rate variability: New perspectives on physiological mechanisms, assessment of self-regulatory capacity, and health risk. *Global Advances in Health and Medicine, 4*(1), 46-61.

(2) Thayer, J. F., Åhs, F., Fredrikson, M., Sollers, J. J., & Wager, T. D. (2012). A meta-analysis of heart rate variability and neuroimaging studies: Implications for heart rate variability as a marker of stress and health. *Neuroscience & Biobehavioral Reviews, 36*(2), 747-756.

(3) Hänsel, A., & von Känel, R. (2008). The ventro-medial prefrontal cortex: A major link between the autonomic nervous system, regulation of emotion, and stress reactivity. *Biopsychosoc Med, 2,* 21.

(4) Elliot, A. J., Payen, V., Brisswalter, J., Cury, F., & Thayer, J. F. (2011). A subtle threat cue, heart rate variability, and cognitive performance. *Psychophysiology*, 48(10), 1340-1345.
(5) Park G., & Thayer, J. F. (2014). From the heart to the mind: Cardiac vagal tone modulates top-down and bottom-up visual perception and attention to emotional stimuli. *Frontiers in Psychology*, 5, 278.

By deliberately slowing the breath we can shift to a calmer state:
(1) Lehrer, P. M. (2007). Biofeedback training to increase heart rate variability. *Principles and Practice of Stress Management*, Third Edition, edited by P.M. Lehrer, R.L. Woolfolk, W.E. Sime, pp. 227-248.
(2) Lin, I. M., Tai, L. Y., & Fan, S. Y. (2014). Breathing at a rate of 5.5 breaths per minute with equal inhalation-to-exhalation ratio increases heart rate variability. *International Journal of Psychophysiology*, 91(3), 206-211.
(3) Jerath, R., Crawford, M. W., Barnes, V. A., & Harden, K. (2015). Self-regulation of breathing as a primary treatment for anxiety. *Applied Psychophysiology and Biofeedback*, 40(2), 107-115.
(4) Lehrer, P. M., & Gevirtz, R. (2014). Heart rate variability biofeedback: How and why does it work?. *Frontiers in Psychology*, 5:756.
(5) Kim, S. H., Schneider, S. M., Bevans, M., Kravitz, L., Mermier, C., Qualls, C., & Burge, M. R. (2013). PTSD symptom reduction with mindfulness-based stretching and deep breathing exercise: Randomized controlled clinical trial of efficacy. *The Journal of Clinical Endocrinology & Metabolism*, 98(7), 2984-2992.

Heart rate variability is linked to self-control:
(1) *Pause-and-plan response:* Segerstrom, S. C., & Nes, L. S. (2007). Heart rate variability reflects self-regulatory strength, effort, and fatigue. *Psychological Science*, 18(3), 275-281.
(2) Hänsel, A., & von Känel, R. (2008). The ventro-medial prefrontal cortex: A major link between the autonomic nervous system, regulation of emotion, and stress reactivity. *Biopsychosoc Med*, 2, 21.

(3) *High-craving alcoholics had lower tonic heart rate variability:* Ingjaldsson, J. T., Thayer, J. F., & Laberg, J. C. (2003). Craving for alcohol and pre-attentive processing of alcohol stimuli. *International Journal of Psychophysiology, 49*(1), 29-39.
(4) Reynard, A., Gevirtz, R., Berlow, R., Brown, M., & Boutelle, K. (2011). Heart rate variability as a marker of self-regulation. *Applied Psychophysiology and Biofeedback, 36*(3), 209-215.

Positive and negative emotions are reflected in the pattern of the heart's rhythm:
(1) Kok, B.E., & Fredrickson. B.L. (2010). Upward spirals of the heart: Autonomic flexibility, as indexed by vagal tone, reciprocally and prospectively predicts positive emotions and social connectedness. *Biological Psychology 85*(3), 432-436.
(2) Shaffer, F., McCraty, R., & Zerr, C. L. (2014). A healthy heart is not a metronome: An integrative review of the heart's anatomy and heart rate variability. *Frontiers in psychology, 5*.

Self-compassion also has a positive effect on HRV: Arch, J. J., Brown, K. W., Dean, D. J., Landy, L. N., Brown, K. D., & Laudenslager, M. L. (2014). Self-compassion training modulates alpha-amylase, heart rate variability, and subjective responses to social evaluative threat in women. *Psychoneuroendocrinology, 42*, 49-58.

HRV biofeedback reduces food cravings: Meule, A., Freund, R., Skirde, A. K., Vögele, C., & Kübler, A. (2012). Heart rate variability biofeedback reduces food cravings in high food cravers. *Applied Psychophysiology and Biofeedback, 37*(4), 241-251.

HRV is associated with weight-loss success and BMI:
(1) Meule, A., Lutz, A., Vögele, C., & Kübler, A. (2012). Self-reported dieting success is associated with cardiac autonomic regulation in current dieters. *Appetite, 59*(2), 494-498.

(2) Koenig, J., Jarczok, M. N., Warth, M., Ellis, R. J., Bach, C., Hillecke, T. K., & Thayer, J. F. (2014). Body mass index is related to autonomic nervous system activity as measured by heart rate variability - a replication using short term measurements. *The Journal of Nutrition, Health & Aging, 18*(3), 300-302.

Physical activity is an excellent way to reduce stress, anxiety, and emotional eating:
(1) Anderson, E., & Shivakumar, G. (2013). Effects of exercise and physical activity on anxiety. *Frontiers in Psychiatry, 4*, 27.
(2) *Obese women completing low/moderate exercise had significant reductions in depression scores*: Annesi, J. J., & Vaughn, L. L. (2011). Relationship of exercise volume with change in depression and its association with self-efficacy to control emotional eating in severely obese women. *Advances in Preventive Medicine, 2011*, 514271.
(3) van Praag, H. (2009). Exercise and the brain: Something to chew on. *Trends in Neurosciences, 32*(5), 283-290.

Exercise counteracts the effects of stress at the cellular level: Puterman, E., Lin, J., Blackburn, E., O'Donovan, A., Adler, N., & Epel, E. (2010). The power of exercise: Buffering the effect of chronic stress on telomere length. *PLoS One, 5*(5), e10837.

Physical activity helps to control body weight:
(1) Ramage, S., Farmer, A., Apps Eccles, K., & McCargar, L. (2013). Healthy strategies for successful weight loss and weight maintenance: A systematic review. *Applied Physiology, Nutrition, and Metabolism, 39*(1), 1-20.
(2) Kilpeläinen, T. O., Qi, L., Brage, S., Sharp, S. J., Sonestedt, E., Demerath, E., ... & Hallmans, G. (2011). Physical activity attenuates the influence of FTO variants on obesity risk: A meta-analysis of 218,166 adults and 19,268 children. *PLoS Medicine, 8*(11), 1543.
(3) *The regular practice of physical activity is associated with weight-loss success*: Annesi, J. J., & Johnson, P. H. (2015). Theory-based psychosocial factors

that discriminate between weight-loss success and failure over 6 months in women with morbid obesity receiving behavioral treatments. *Eating and Weight Disorders-Studies on Anorexia, Bulimia and Obesity*, 20(2), 223-232.

79% of Americans don't meet exercise guidelines: Harris, C.D., Watson, K.B., Carlson, S.A., Fulton, J.E., Dorn, J.M., & Elam-Evans, L. (2013). Adult participation in aerobic and muscle-strengthening physical activities — United States, 2011. *Morbidity and Mortality Weekly Report* 62(17), 326-330.

Physical activity diminishes reward-driven eating:
(1) Killgore, W. D., Kipman, M., Schwab, Z. J., Tkachenko, O., Preer, L., Gogel, H., ... & Weber, M. (2013). Physical exercise and brain responses to images of high-calorie food. *Neuroreport, 24*(17), 962-967.
(2) Joseph, R. J., Alonso-Alonso, M., Bond, D. S., Pascual-Leone, A., & Blackburn, G. L. (2011). The neurocognitive connection between physical activity and eating behaviour. *Obesity Reviews, 12*(10), 800-812.
(3) *Exercise reduces urges for sugary snacks:* Ledochowski, L., Ruedl, G., Taylor, A. H., & Kopp, M. (2015). Acute effects of brisk walking on sugary snack cravings in overweight people, affect and responses to a manipulated stress situation and to a sugary snack cue: A crossover study. *PloS One, 10*(3), e0119278.

Exercise for mood and anxiety: Otto, M., & Smits, J. A. (2011). *Exercise for Mood and Anxiety: Proven Strategies for Overcoming Depression and Enhancing Well-Being*. Oxford: Oxford University Press.

Just start with a 15 minute walk:
(1) *Positive responses are experienced after relatively short bouts of acute exercise*: Daley, A. J., & Welch, A. (2004). The effects of 15 min and 30 min of exercise on affective responses both during and after exercise. *Journal of Sports Sciences, 22*(7), 621-628.
(2) *Health benefits are seen with 30 minutes daily*: Hansen, C. J., Stevens, L. C., & Coast, J. R. (2001). Exercise duration and mood state: How much is enough to feel better? *Health Psychology, 20*(4), 267.

(3) *Long term weight-loss is associated with longer exercise periods (~1 hr/day):* Wing, R. R., & Phelan, S. (2005). Long-term weight loss maintenance. *The American Journal of Clinical Nutrition, 82*(1), 222S-225S.

To form a habit, repeat an action consistently in the same context: Gardner, B., Lally, P., & Wardle, J. (2012). Making health habitual: The psychology of 'habit-formation'and general practice. *British Journal of General Practice, 62*(605), 664-666.

It takes months to change longstanding habits: Lally, P., Van Jaarsveld, C. H., Potts, H. W., & Wardle, J. (2010). How are habits formed: Modelling habit formation in the real world. *European Journal of Social Psychology, 40*(6), 998-1009.

Actions that are initially difficult to stick to become easier to maintain and they ultimately become second nature: Lally, P., Wardle, J., & Gardner, B. (2011). Experiences of habit formation: A qualitative study. *Psychology, Health & Medicine, 16*(4), 484-489.

CHAPTER 11. DELAY GRATIFICATION
A competition between "hot" and "cool" systems:
(1) Metcalfe, J., & Mischel, W. (1999). A hot/cool-system analysis of delay of gratification: Dynamics of willpower. *Psychological Review, 106*(1), 3.
(2) Hofmann, W., Friese, M., & Strack, F. (2009). Impulse and self-control from a dual-systems perspective. *Perspectives on Psychological Science, 4*(2), 162-176.
(3) He, Q., Xiao, L., Xue, G., Wong, S., Ames, S. L., Schembre, S. M., & Bechara, A. (2014). Poor ability to resist tempting calorie rich food is linked to altered balance between neural systems involved in urge and self-control. *Nutrition Journal, 13*(1), 92.
(4) Bechara, A. (2005). Decision making, impulse control and loss of will-power to resist drugs: A neurocognitive perspective. *Nature Neuroscience, 8*(11), 1458-1463.

Delay automatic responses until the "hot" signal subsides: *Self-control requires individuals to delay behavior until sufficient pre-action information processing has occurred. Instead of listening to common wisdom and "fighting" your urges by "exerting" your willpower to counter a temptation, you may fare much better by simply relaxing and adopting a goal to be inactive:* Hepler, J., Albarracin, D., McCulloch, K. C., & Noguchi, K. (2012). Being active and impulsive: The role of goals for action and inaction in self-control. *Motivation and Emotion, 36*(4), 416-424.

The Marshmallow Test:
(1) Mischel W., Shoda, Y., & Rodriguez, M. I. (1989). Delay of gratification in children. *Science, 244*(4907), 933-938.
(2) Mischel, W., Ph.D. (2014). *The Marshmallow Test: Mastering Self Control.* (New York: Little, Brown and Company), p. 248.

Delayed gratification in childhood, link to BMI: Schlam, T. R., Wilson, N. L., Shoda, Y., Mischel, W., & Ayduk, O. (2013). Preschoolers' delay of gratification predicts their body mass 30 years later. *The Journal of Pediatrics, 162*(1), 90-93.

Dr. Walter Mischel: *Use the "cool" system to cognitively reappraise temptations, and activate the "hot" system to make representations of the future more powerful:* p. 248 in Mischel, W., Ph.D. (2014). *The marshmallow test: Mastering self-control.* New York: Little, Brown and Company.

Focusing on the long-term consequences of unhealthy food makes it less desirable:
(1) Hollands, G. J., Prestwich, A., & Marteau, T. M. (2011). Using aversive images to enhance healthy food choices and implicit attitudes: An experimental test of evaluative conditioning. *Health Psychology, 30*(2), 195.
(2) Hofmann, W., Deutsch, R., Lancaster, K., & Banaji, M. R. (2010). Cooling the heat of temptation: Mental self-control and the automatic

evaluation of tempting stimuli. *European Journal of Social Psychology*, *40*(1), 17-25.

(3) *Cognitive reappraisal significantly decreases cravings for hyperpalatable foods*: Giuliani, N. R., Calcott, R. D., & Berkman, E. T. (2013). Piece of cake: Cognitive reappraisal of food craving. *Appetite, 64*, 56-61.

(4) Dassen, F. C., Houben, K., & Jansen, A. (2015). Time orientation and eating behavior: Unhealthy eaters consider immediate consequences, while healthy eaters focus on future health. *Appetite*, 91, 13-19.

Physical activity improves mood and self-efficacy:

(1) *Increasing physical activity volume was associated with higher levels of happiness*: Richards, J., Jiang, X., Kelly, P., Chau, J., Bauman, A., & Ding, D. (2015). Don't worry, be happy: Cross-sectional associations between physical activity and happiness in 15 European countries. *BMC Public Health*, *15*(1), 53.

(2) *Low/moderate exercise helped reduce depression, increase self-efficacy*: Annesi, J. J., & Vaughn, L. L. (2011). Relationship of exercise volume with change in depression and its association with self-efficacy to control emotional eating in severely obese women. *Advances in Preventive Medicine, 2011*, 514271.

Mindfulness and resonant breathing activate the pause-and-plan response:

(1) *Enhanced attention to present experiences can strengthen the link between intentions and behavior*: Chatzisarantis, N. L., & Hagger, M. S. (2007). Mindfulness and the intention-behavior relationship within the theory of planned behavior. *Personality and Social Psychology Bulletin, 33*(5), 663-676.

(2) Segerstrom, S. C., & Nes, L. S. (2007). Heart rate variability reflects self-regulatory strength, effort, and fatigue. *Psychological Science, 18*(3), 275-281.

(3) Reynard, A., Gevirtz, R., Berlow, R., Brown, M., & Boutelle, K. (2011). Heart rate variability as a marker of self-regulation. *Applied Psychophysiology and Biofeedback, 36*(3), 209-215.

Self-compassion counteracts black-and white thinking:
(1) *Self–compassion modulates the "what-the-hell" effect*: Adams, C. E., & Leary, M. R. (2007). Promoting self-compassionate attitudes toward eating among restrictive and guilty eaters. *Journal of Social and Clinical Psychology, 26*(10), 1120-1144.
(2) *A mindfulness plus self-compassion group lost more weight*: Mantzios, M., & Wilson, J. C. (2014). Exploring mindfulness and mindfulness with self-compassion-centered interventions to assist weight loss: Theoretical considerations and preliminary results of a randomized pilot study. *Mindfulness,* July 2014, 1-12.
(3) Inzlicht, M., Legault, L., & Teper, R. (2014). Exploring the mechanisms of self-control improvement. *Current Directions in Psychological Science, 23*(4), 302-307.

Use implementation intentions in order to persist with your goals:
(1) Koestner, R., Lekes, N., Powers, T. A., & Chicoine, E. (2002). Attaining personal goals: Self-concordance plus implementation intentions equals success. *Journal of Personality and Social Psychology, 83*(1), 231.
(2) Gollwitzer, P. M., & Schaal, B. (1998). Metacognition in action: The importance of implementation intentions. *Personality and Social Psychology Review, 2*(2), 124-136.
(3) Hattar, A., Hagger, M. S., & Pal, S. (2015). Weight-loss intervention using implementation intentions and mental imagery: A randomized control trial study protocol. *BMC Public Health, 15*(1), 196.

Prepare and plan meals with tasty, nutrient-dense foods: Conner, T. S., Brookie, K. L., Richardson, A. C., & Polak, M. A. (2015). On carrots and curiosity: Eating fruit and vegetables is associated with greater flourishing in daily life. *British Journal of Health Psychology, 20*(2), 413-427.

The joy of trying new tastes: *Adventurous eating could help individuals lose/maintain weight without feeling as restricted. Individuals who are willing to try new nutrient-dense foods have lower BMIs:* Latimer, L. A., Pope, L.,

& Wansink, B. (2015). Food neophiles: Profiling the adventurous eater. Obesity, 23(8), 1577-1581.

Every instance of successful planning and implementation contributes to short-term satisfaction (and long-term success):
(1) *People high in self-control experience higher levels of momentary affect even as they experience desire:* Hofmann, W., Luhmann, M., Fisher, R. R., Vohs, K. D., & Baumeister, R. F. (2014). Yes, but are they happy? Effects of trait self-control on affective well-being and life satisfaction. *Journal of Personality, 82*(4), 265-277.
(2) *Individual momentary happiness can be maximized by avoiding temptations altogether:* Hofmann, W., Kotabe, H., & Luhmann, M. (2013). The spoiled pleasure of giving in to temptation. Motivation and Emotion, 37(4), 733-742.

CHAPTER 12. FOCUS ON NUTRIENT-DENSE FOODS
Nutrient-dense foods:
(1) *The Nutrient Rich Foods Index emphasizes nutrient density, defined as nutrients per calorie:* Drewnowski, A. (2010). The Nutrient Rich Foods Index helps to identify healthy, affordable foods. *The American Journal of Clinical Nutrition, 91*(4), 1095S-1101S.
(2) *"Powerhouse" fruits and vegetables have been defined as foods providing, on average, 10% or more daily value per 100 kcal of 17 qualifying nutrients:* Di Noia, J. (2014). Defining powerhouse fruits and vegetables: A nutrient density approach. *Preventing Chronic Disease, 11,*130390.
(3) *Long-term weight control is associated with the intake of vegetables, whole grains, fruits, nuts, and yogurt:* Mozaffarian, D., Hao, T., Rimm, E. B., Willett, W. C., & Hu, F. B. (2011). Changes in diet and lifestyle and long-term weight gain in women and men. *New England Journal of Medicine, 364*(25), 2392-2404.
(4) *Successful weight-loss maintainers ate more vegetables and whole grains:* Raynor, H. A., Van Walleghen, E. L., Bachman, J. L., Looney, S. M., Phelan, S., & Wing, R. R. (2011). Dietary energy density and successful weight loss maintenance. *Eating Behaviors, 12*(2), 119-125.

Sugar squeezes nutrients out of the diet: Marriott, B. P., Olsho, L., Hadden, L., & Connor, P. (2010). Intake of added sugars and selected nutrients in the United States, National Health and Nutrition Examination Survey (NHANES) 2003—2006. *Critical Reviews in Food Science and Nutrition*, *50*(3), 228-258.

Aim for 30 minutes of moderate physical activity daily: American Heart Association. (2015). American Heart Association recommendations for physical activity in adults. Retrieved from <http://www.heart.org/ HEARTORG/GettingHealthy/PhysicalActivity/FitnessBasics/American-Heart-Association-Recommendations-for-Physical-Activity-in-Adults_ UCM_307976_Article.jsp>

The average U.S. diet contains too many calories, not enough nutrients: (1) U.S. Department of Health and Human Services. Scientific Report of the 2015 Dietary Guidelines Advisory Committee, Part D, Chapter 1: Food and nutrient intakes and health: Current status and trends - Nutrient intake and nutrients of concern. Retrieved from <http://www. health.gov/dietaryguidelines/2015-scientific-report/06-chapter-1/ d1-2.asp>
(2) U.S. Department of Agriculture. Report of the Dietary Guidelines Advisory Committee on the Dietary Guidelines for Americans, 2010. Retrieved from <http://origin.www.cnpp.usda.gov/DGAs2010-DGACReport.htm>
(3) *Fewer than 1 in 10 Americans meet fruit or vegetable recommendations*: Kimmons, J., Gillespie, C., Seymour, J., Serdula, M., & Blanck, H. M. (2009). Fruit and vegetable intake among adolescents and adults in the United States: Percentage meeting individualized recommendations. *The Medscape Journal of Medicine*, *11*(1), 26.
(4) The Academy of Nutrition and Dietetics. (2015). Dietary guidelines and MyPlate. Retrieved from <http://www.eatright.org/resources/food/ nutrition/dietary-guidelines-and-myplate>

A majority of respondents were unable to identify their nutritional requirements:
(1) Epstein, S. B., Jean-Pierre, K., Lynn, S., & Kant, A. K. (2013). Media coverage and awareness of the 2010 Dietary Guidelines for Americans and MyPlate. *American Journal of Health Promotion, 28*(1), e30-e39.
(2) International Food Information Council Foundation. (2012). 2012 Food & Health Survey: Consumer Attitudes toward Food Safety, Nutrition and Health. Updated November 7, 2014. Retrieved from <http://www.foodinsight.org/2012_Food_Health_Survey_Consumer_Attitudes_toward_Food_Safety_Nutrition_and_Health#sthash.8vf3VCge.dpuf>
(3) *As of 2012, only 16% of U.S. medical schools required a dedicated nutrition course*: DiMaria-Ghalili, R. A., Edwards, M., Friedman, G., Jaferi, A., Kohlmeier, M., Kris-Etherton, P., ... & Wylie-Rosett, J. (2013). Capacity building in nutrition science: Revisiting the curricula for medical professionals. *Annals of the New York Academy of Sciences, 1306*(1), 21-40.

American Heart Association recommendations: The American Heart Association's Diet and Lifestyle Recommendations. June 10, 2015. Retrieved from <http://www.heart.org/HEARTORG/GettingHealthy/NutritionCenter/HealthyEating/The-American-Heart-Associations-Diet-and-Lifestyle-Recommendations_UCM_305855_Article.jsp>

Harvard School of Public Health recommendations: Healthy eating plate and healthy eating pyramid. (2011). For more information about The Healthy Eating Plate, see The Nutrition Source, Department of Nutrition, Harvard School of Public Health, www.thenutritionsource.org, and Harvard Health Publications, www.health.harvard.edu.

Mayo Clinic recommendations: Nutrition and Healthy Eating. (2014). Retrieved from <http://www.mayoclinic.org/healthy-lifestyle/nutrition-and-healthy-eating/basics/healthy-diets/hlv-20049477>

Many eating patterns can work:
(1) Freeland-Graves, J. H., & Nitzke, S. (2013). Position of the Academy of Nutrition and Dietetics: Total diet approach to healthy eating. *Journal of the Academy of Nutrition and Dietetics, 113*(2), 307-317.
(2) *Reduced-calorie diets result in weight loss regardless of which macronutrients they emphasize:* Sacks, F. M., Bray, G. A., Carey, V. J., Smith, S. R., Ryan, D. H., Anton, S. D., ... & Leboff, M. S. (2009). Comparison of weight-loss diets with different compositions of fat, protein, and carbohydrates. *New England Journal of Medicine, 360*(9), 859-873.
(3) *Weight loss differences between individual named diets were small. This supports the practice of recommending any diet that a patient will adhere to in order to lose weight:* Johnston, B. C., Kanters, S., Bandayrel, K., Wu, P., Naji, F., Siemieniuk, R. A., ... & Jansen, J. P. (2014). Comparison of weight loss among named diet programs in overweight and obese adults: A meta-analysis. *JAMA, 312*(9), 923-933.
(4) *Behavioral adherence is more important than diet composition. The assumption that one diet is optimal for all persons is counterproductive:* Pagoto, S. L., & Appelhans, B. M. (2013). A call for an end to the diet debates. *JAMA, 310*(7), 687-688.
(5) *At the end of the day it is the diet you can stick to that will be the perfect diet for you:* Pagoto, S. L. (2013). The perfect diet doesn't exist. August 20, 2013. Retrieved from <http://www.fudiet.com/2013/08/the-perfect-diet-doesnt-exist/>

What about sugar? World Health Organization. (2015). WHO calls on countries to reduce sugars intake among adults and children. Press release, March 4, 2015. Retrieved from <http://www.who.int/mediacentre/news/releases/2015/sugar-guideline/en/>

Although many dieters go for calorie-free sodas, there is growing concern:
(1) *Households purchasing more than twenty 12-packs of diet soda annually generally purchase more snack foods at the grocery store and more overall calories:*

Bleich, S. N., Wolfson, J. A., Vine, S., & Wang, Y. C. (2014). Diet-beverage consumption and caloric intake among US adults, overall and by body weight. *American Journal of Public Health*, *104*(3), e72-e78.
(2) *Some artificial sweeteners may alter the gut microbiota*: Suez, J., Korem, T., Zeevi, D., Zilberman-Schapira, G., Thaiss, C. A., Maza, O., ... & Elinav, E. (2014). Artificial sweeteners induce glucose intolerance by altering the gut microbiota. *Nature*, *514*(7521), 181-186.
(3) *Cola products are associated with bone mineral loss*: Tucker, K. L., Morita, K., Qiao, N., Hannan, M. T., Cupples, L. A., & Kiel, D. P. (2006). Colas, but not other carbonated beverages, are associated with low bone mineral density in older women: The Framingham Osteoporosis Study. *The American Journal of Clinical Nutrition*, *84*(4), 936-942.

The American Heart Association suggests using a small amount of sugar if needed to improve the taste of healthy foods: American Heart Association, Getting Healthy, Nutrition Center. Sugar 101. Updated Nov 19, 2014. Retrieved from <http://www.heart.org/HEARTORG/GettingHealthy/ NutritionCenter/Sugars-101_UCM_306024_Article.jsp>

Stevia is a natural calorie-free sweetener:
(1) Lemus-Mondaca, R., Vega-Gálvez, A., Zura-Bravo, L., & Ah-Hen, K. (2012*). Stevia rebaudiana* Bertoni, source of a high-potency natural sweetener: A comprehensive review on the biochemical, nutritional and functional aspects. *Food Chemistry*, *132*(3), 1121-1132.
(2) *Stevia provides a level of satiety similar to that of sucrose*: Anton, S. D., Martin, C. K., Han, H., Coulon, S., Cefalu, W. T., Geiselman, P., & Williamson, D. A. (2010). Effects of stevia, aspartame, and sucrose on food intake, satiety, and postprandial glucose and insulin levels. *Appetite*, *55*(1), 37-43.

A plant-based diet can lower cholesterol: Ferdowsian, H. R., & Barnard, N. D. (2009). Effects of plant-based diets on plasma lipids. *The American Journal of Cardiology*, *104*(7), 947.

Dr. Dean Ornish: Ornish, D., & Brown, S. E. (2002). *Eat More, Weigh Less: Dr. Dean Ornish's Program for Losing Weight Safely While Eating Abundantly.* New York: HarperTorch.

Omega-3 fatty acids:
(1) Jump, D. B., Depner, C. M., & Tripathy, S. (2012). Omega-3 fatty acid supplementation and cardiovascular disease Thematic Review Series: New lipid and lipoprotein targets for the treatment of cardiometabolic diseases. *Journal of Lipid Research, 53*(12), 2525-2545.
(2) Swanson, D., Block, R., & Mousa, S. A. (2012). Omega-3 fatty acids EPA and DHA: Health benefits throughout life. *Advances in Nutrition: An International Review Journal, 3*(1), 1-7.
(3) Jain, A. P., Aggarwal, K. K., & Zhang, P. Y. (2015). Omega-3 fatty acids and cardiovascular disease. *Eur Rev Med Pharmacol Sci, 19*(3), 441-5.

Yogurt for good health:
(1) Wang, H., Livingston, K. A., Fox, C. S., Meigs, J. B., & Jacques, P. F. (2013). Yogurt consumption is associated with better diet quality and metabolic profile in American men and women. *Nutrition Research, 33*(1), 18-26.
(2) Webb, D., Donovan, S. M., & Meydani, S. N. (2014). The role of yogurt in improving the quality of the American diet and meeting dietary guidelines. *Nutrition Reviews, 72*(3), 180-189.
(3) Lourens-Hattingh, A., & Viljoen, B. C. (2001). Yogurt as probiotic carrier food. *International Dairy Journal, 11*(1), 1-17.
(4) National Yogurt Association website. <http://www.aboutyogurt.com/>

The balance of bacteria may help protect against obesity:
(1) Okeke, F., Roland, B. C., & Mullin, G. E. (2014). The role of the gut microbiome in the pathogenesis and treatment of obesity. *Global Advances in Health and Medicine, 3*(3), 44-57.
(2) Poutahidis, T., Kleinewietfeld, M., Smillie, C., Levkovich, T., Perrotta, A., Bhela, S., ... & Erdman, S. E. (2013). Microbial reprogramming inhibits Western diet-associated obesity. *PLoS One, 8*(7), e68596.

Kefir as a source of probiotic bacteria:
(1) Turan, İ., Dedeli, Ö., Bor, S., & İlter, T. (2014). Effects of a kefir supplement on symptoms, colonic transit, and bowel satisfaction score in patients with chronic constipation: A pilot study. *The Turkish Journal of Gastroenterology: The Official Journal of Turkish Society of Gastroenterology*, *25*(6), 650-656.
(2) Leite, A. M. D. O., Miguel, M. A. L., Peixoto, R. S., Rosado, A. S., Silva, J. T., & Paschoalin, V. M. F. (2013). Microbiological, technological and therapeutic properties of kefir: A natural probiotic beverage. *Brazilian Journal of Microbiology*, *44*(2), 341-349.

Gut bifidobacteria contribute to good health:
(1) Yang, H. Y., Liu, S. L., Ibrahim, S. A., Zhao, L., Jiang, J. L., Sun, W. F., & Ren, F. Z. (2009). Oral administration of live *Bifidobacterium* substrains isolated from healthy centenarians enhanced immune function in BALB/c mice. *Nutrition Research*, *29*(4), 281-289.
(2) Biagi, E., Nylund, L., Candela, M., Ostan, R., Bucci, L., Pini, E., ... & De Vos, W. (2010). Through ageing, and beyond: Gut microbiota and inflammatory status in seniors and centenarians. *PLoS One*, *5*(5), e10667.
(3) Arunachalam, K., Gill, H. S., & Chandra, R. K. (2000). Enhancement of natural immune function by dietary consumption of *Bifidobacterium lactis* (HN019). *European Journal of Clinical Nutrition*, *54*(3), 263-267.
(4) Selhub, E. M., Logan, A. C., & Bested, A. C. (2014). Fermented foods, microbiota, and mental health: Ancient practice meets nutritional psychiatry. *Journal of Physiological Anthropology*, *33*(1), 1.

Probiotic bacteria may ameliorate irritable bowel syndrome:
(1) Kennedy, P. J., Cryan, J. F., Dinan, T. G., & Clarke, G. (2014). Irritable bowel syndrome: A microbiome-gut-brain axis disorder? *World Journal of Gastroenterology: WJG*, *20*(39), 14105.
(2) Didari, T., Mozaffari, S., Nikfar, S., & Abdollahi, M. (2015). Effectiveness of probiotics in irritable bowel syndrome: Updated systematic review with meta-analysis. *World Journal of Gastroenterology: WJG*, *21*(10), 3072.

(3) Yoon, H., Park, Y. S., Lee, D. H., Seo, J. G., Shin, C. M., & Kim, N. (2015). Effect of administering a multi-species probiotic mixture on the changes in fecal microbiota and symptoms of irritable bowel syndrome: A randomized, double-blind, placebo-controlled trial. *Journal of Clinical Biochemistry and Nutrition, 57*(2), 129.

Probiotics may boost immunity and reduce inflammation: Drisko, J. A., Giles, C. K., & Bischoff, B. J. (2003). Probiotics in health maintenance and disease prevention. *Alternative Medicine Review, 8*(2), 143-155.

Lactose intolerance: *The bacteria inherent in yogurt assist in digesting lactose*: Savaiano, D. A. (2014). Lactose digestion from yogurt: Mechanism and relevance. *The American Journal of Clinical Nutrition, 99*(5), 1251S-1255S.

Dietary fiber reduces the risk of many chronic diseases:
(1) Anderson, J. W., Baird, P., Davis, R. H., Ferreri, S., Knudtson, M., Koraym, A., ... & Williams, C. L. (2009). Health benefits of dietary fiber. *Nutrition Reviews, 67*(4), 188-205.
(2) Slavin, J. (2013). Fiber and prebiotics: Mechanisms and health benefits. *Nutrients, 5*(4), 1417-1435.
(3) Mobley, A. R., Jones, J. M., Rodriguez, J., Slavin, J., & Zelman, K. M. (2014). Identifying practical solutions to meet America's fiber needs: Proceedings from the Food & Fiber Summit. *Nutrients, 6*(7), 2540-2551.
(4) Riccardi, G., Rivellese, A. A., & Giacco, R. (2008). Role of glycemic index and glycemic load in the healthy state, in prediabetes, and in diabetes. *The American Journal of Clinical Nutrition, 87*(1), 269S-274S.

Dietary fiber intake is currently inadequate:
(1) Mobley, A. R., Slavin, J. L., & Hornick, B. A. (2013). The future of recommendations on grain foods in dietary guidance. *The Journal of Nutrition, 143*(9), 1527S-1532S.

(2) U.S. Department of Agriculture, Agricultural Research Service. (2010). What we eat in America. Nutrient intakes from food, NHANES 2007–2008; Technical Report, 2010. Retrieved from < http://www.ars.usda.gov/ main/main.htm >

Dietary Guidelines, MyPlate: U.S. Department of Agriculture. Choose My Plate. Retrieved from <http://www.choosemyplate.gov/about.html>

Fiber promotes weight loss (Dr. Susan Roberts): US Department of Agriculture. (2015). Shifting out of high-calorie habits. Agricultural Research Magazine, March 2015. Retrieved from <http://agresearchmag. ars.usda.gov/2015/mar/calories/>

The Harvard School of Public Health encourages us to limit red meat and avoid processed meats: Harvard T.H. Chan School of Public Health, Harvard University. (2011). Healthy Eating Plate & Healthy Eating Pyramid. Retrieved from < http://www.hsph.harvard.edu/nutritionsource/ healthy-eating-plate/>

What about wheat:
(1) Gaesser, G. A., & Angadi, S. S. (2012). Gluten-free diet: Imprudent dietary advice for the general population?. *Journal of the Academy of Nutrition and Dietetics, 112*(9), 1330-1333.
(2) Kent, P. S. (2013). Is going gluten free the next fad diet?. Journal of Renal Nutrition, 23(2), e47-e50.

The consumption of dairy products and calcium is associated with a decreased risk of obesity:
(1) Zemel, M. B., Thompson, W., Milstead, A., Morris, K., & Campbell, P. (2004). Calcium and dairy acceleration of weight and fat loss during energy restriction in obese adults. *Obesity Research, 12*(4), 582-590.
(2) Murphy, K. J., Crichton, G. E., Dyer, K. A., Coates, A. M., Pettman, T. L., Milte, C., ... & Howe, P. R. (2013). Dairy foods and dairy protein

consumption is inversely related to markers of adiposity in obese men and women. *Nutrients*, *5*(11), 4665-4684.

(3) Abargouei, A. S., Janghorbani, M., Salehi-Marzijarani, M., & Esmaillzadeh, A. (2012). Effect of dairy consumption on weight and body composition in adults: A systematic review and meta-analysis of randomized controlled clinical trials. *International Journal of Obesity*, *36*(12), 1485-1493.

(4) Keast, D. R., Gallant, K. M. H., Albertson, A. M., Gugger, C. K., & Holschuh, N. M. (2015). Associations between yogurt, dairy, calcium, and Vitamin D intake and obesity among U.S. children aged 8–18 years: NHANES, 2005–2008. *Nutrients*, *7*(3), 1577-1593.

Don't drink your calories, just drink water:

(1) *Dieters who drank water before meals lost more weight:* Dennis, E. A., Dengo, A. L., Comber, D. L., Flack, K. D., Savla, J., Davy, K. P., & Davy, B. M. (2010). Water consumption increases weight loss during a hypocaloric diet intervention in middle-aged and older adults. *Obesity*, *18*(2), 300-307.

(2) *Beverages containing calories contribute extra calories in a near-additive fashion*: Appelhans, B. M., Bleil, M. E., Waring, M. E., Schneider, K. L., Nackers, L. M., Busch, A. M., ... & Pagoto, S. L. (2013). Beverages contribute extra calories to meals and daily energy intake in overweight and obese women. *Physiology & Behavior*, *122*, 129-133.

(3) *Juice does not produce satiety*: Flood-Obbagy, J. E., & Rolls, B. J. (2009). The effect of fruit in different forms on energy intake and satiety at a meal. *Appetite*, *52*(2), 416-422.

(4) Hu, F. B. (2013). Resolved: There is sufficient scientific evidence that decreasing sugar-sweetened beverage consumption will reduce the prevalence of obesity and obesity-related diseases. *Obesity Reviews*, 14(8), 606-619.

(5) *Those who drink alcohol tend to gain weight*: Jung, S. Y., Vitolins, M. Z., Fenton, J., Frazier-Wood, A. C., Hursting, S. D., & Chang, S. (2015). Risk

profiles for weight gain among postmenopausal women: A classification and regression tree analysis approach. *PloS One, 10*(3).

It is important to consume regular meals in the same place and at the same time of day:
(1) *Focus on doing one thing in a consistent context*: Gardner, B., Lally, P., & Wardle, J. (2012). Making health habitual: The psychology of 'habit-formation' and general practice. *British Journal of General Practice, 62*(605), 664-666.
(2) *The importance of three meals per day*: Leidy, H. J., & Campbell, W. W. (2011). The effect of eating frequency on appetite control and food intake: brief synopsis of controlled feeding studies. *The Journal of Nutrition, 141*(1), 154-157.
(3) *Successful weight maintenance is associated with a regular meal rhythm*: Elfhag, K., & Rössner, S. (2005). Who succeeds in maintaining weight loss? A conceptual review of factors associated with weight loss maintenance and weight regain. *Obesity Reviews, 6*(1), 67-85.
(4) *The importance of establishing a regular daily lifestyle*: Tighe, C. A., Dautovich, N. D., & Allen, R. S. (2015). Regularity of daily activities buffers the negative impact of low perceived control on affect. *Motivation and Emotion, 39*(3), 448-457.
(5) *Greater meal regularity is associated with greater weight loss*: Fuglestad, P. T., Jeffery, R. W., & Sherwood, N. E. (2012). Lifestyle patterns associated with diet, physical activity, body mass index and amount of recent weight loss in a sample of successful weight losers. *Int J Behav Nutr Phys Act, 9*(1), 79.

Questions before you eat: Protein requirements depend on your age, gender, and level of physical activity. For protein, fiber, and other nutritional recommendations based on the 2015-2020 Dietary Guidelines see: <http://health.gov/dietaryguidelines/2015/guidelines/appendix-7/>.
For food guidelines see ChooseMyPlate at <http://www.choosemyplate.gov>

CHAPTER 13. SEEK HAPPINESS.

How to experience more happiness in your life:
(1) Ryff, C. D., & Singer, B. H. (2008). Know thyself and become what you are: A eudaimonic approach to psychological well-being. *Journal of Happiness Studies, 9*(1), 13-39.
(2) *This article distinguishes between hedonic and eudaimonic approaches to wellness, with the former focusing on the* outcome *of happiness or pleasure and the latter focusing on the* process *of living well*: Ryan, R. M., Huta, V., & Deci, E. L. (2008). Living well: A self-determination theory perspective on eudaimonia. *Journal of Happiness Studies, 9*(1), 139-170.
(3) *Just as the satisfaction of one's physiological needs (e.g., hunger) is critical for one's physical survival, the satisfaction of one's basic psychological needs is critical for well-being*: Verstuyf, J., Patrick, H., Vansteenkiste, M., & Teixeira, P. J. (2012). Motivational dynamics of eating regulation: A self-determination theory perspective. *International Journal of Behavioral Nutrition and Physical Activity, 9*(1), 1-16.
(4) *Well-being has multiple dimensions, including environmental mastery and autonomy*: Ryff, C. D., & Keyes, C. L. M. (1995). The structure of psychological well-being revisited. *Journal of Personality and Social Psychology, 69*(4), 719.

Weight loss boosts self-confidence and mood:
(1) *Weight loss was associated with lowered depression and increased self-esteem*: Blaine, B. E., Rodman, J., & Newman, J. M. (2007). Weight loss treatment and psychological well-being a review and meta-analysis. *Journal of Health Psychology, 12*(1), 66-82.
(2) *Weight loss led to improvements in energy, physical mobility, general mood, self-confidence, and physical health*: Klem, M. L., Wing, R. R., McGuire, M. T., Seagle, H. M., & Hill, J. O. (1997). A descriptive study of individuals successful at long-term maintenance of substantial weight loss. *The American Journal of Clinical Nutrition, 66*(2), 239-246.
(3) *Weight loss was associated with psychological well-being and vitality*: Swencionis, C., Wylie-Rosett, J., Lent, M. R., Ginsberg, M., Cimino, C.,

Wassertheil-Smoller, S., ... & Segal-Isaacson, C. J. (2013). Weight change, psychological well-being, and vitality in adults participating in a cognitive–behavioral weight loss program. *Health Psychology, 32*(4), 439.

Physical activity contributes to happiness in the short term and long term:
(1) *Physical activity is associated with higher levels of happiness*: Richards, J., Jiang, X., Kelly, P., Chau, J., Bauman, A., & Ding, D. (2015). Don't worry, be happy: Cross-sectional associations between physical activity and happiness in 15 European countries. *BMC Public Health, 15*(1), 53.
(2) Wang, F., Orpana, H. M., Morrison, H., De Groh, M., Dai, S., & Luo, W. (2012). Long-term association between leisure-time physical activity and changes in happiness: Analysis of the Prospective National Population Health Survey. American journal of epidemiology, 176(12), 1095-1100.

Mindfulness and self-compassion contribute to happiness:
(1) Brown, K. W., & Ryan, R. M. (2003). The benefits of being present: Mindfulness and its role in psychological well-being. *Journal of Personality and Social Psychology, 84*(4), 822.
(2) Garland, E. L., Geschwind, N., Peeters, F., & Wichers, M. (2015). Mindfulness training promotes upward spirals of positive affect and cognition: Multilevel and autoregressive latent trajectory modeling analyses. *Frontiers in Psychology, 6*, 15.
(3) Desbordes, G., Gard, T., Hoge, E. A., Hölzel, B. K., Kerr, C., Lazar, S. W., ... & Vago, D. R. (2014). Moving beyond mindfulness: Defining equanimity as an outcome measure in meditation and contemplative research. *Mindfulness, 6*(2), 356-372.
(4) *Mindfulness adds clarity and vividness to current experience:* Brown, K. W., Ryan, R. M., & Creswell, J. D. (2007). Mindfulness: Theoretical foundations and evidence for its salutary effects. *Psychological Inquiry, 18*(4), 211-237.
(5) *People can increase their happiness through simple intentional positive activities, such as expressing gratitude or practicing kindness:* Lyubomirsky, S., & Layous, K. (2013). How do simple positive activities increase well-being?. *Current Directions in Psychological Science, 22*(1), 57-62.

Cognitive reappraisal of events is important for happiness: *Positive reappraisal involves coping with adverse life events with thoughts such as "I think I can learn something from the situation"*: Garland, E., Gaylord, S., & Park, J. (2009). The role of mindfulness in positive reappraisal. *Explore: The Journal of Science and Healing, 5*(1), 37-44.

Self-regulation is concerned with setting goals, developing and enacting strategies to achieve those goals, appraising progress, and revising goals and strategies accordingly: Inzlicht, M., Legault, L., & Teper, R. (2014). Exploring the mechanisms of self-control improvement. *Current Directions in Psychological Science, 23*(4), 302-307.

Self-regulation ability boosts happiness:
(1) *People can enhance their happiness through intentional strategies, such as pursuing personally concordant goals*: Cheung, T. T., Gillebaart, M., Kroese, F., & De Ridder, D. (2014). Why are people with high self-control happier? The effect of trait self-control on happiness as mediated by regulatory focus. *Frontiers in Psychology, 5*. 722.
(2) *Competence (seeking to control the outcome and experience mastery) and autonomy (the universal urge to be causal agents of one's own life and act in harmony with one's integrated self) contribute to psychological well-being*: Ryan, R.M., & Deci, E.L. (2000). Self-determination theory and the facilitation of intrinsic motivation, social development, and well-being. *American Psychologist, 55*, 68–78.

Smokers were never happier than when they were being successful: *Conventional wisdom says that smokers use cigarettes to ease anxiety and depression. However, researchers studied people who were trying to quit and found that they were never happier than when they were being successful, for however long that was*: Kahler, C. W., Spillane, N. S., Busch, A. M., & Leventhal, A. M. (2010). Time-varying smoking abstinence predicts lower depressive symptoms following smoking cessation treatment. *Nicotine & Tobacco Research*, ntq213.

Made in the USA
Lexington, KY
11 September 2016